HOMEOPATHY
MEDICINE THAT
WORKS!

A promise to the reader . . .

- How and why homeopathy works, what it costs, how long it takes, its drawbacks, what it CAN'T cure (e.g. obesity & baldness), its cure rate (about 85%), why it's suddenly so popular—everything you need to know to evaluate it.

Professional care for chronic conditions:

- What it's like to be treated homeopathically, after reading dozens of lively entertaining cured cases.

- How 'constitutional' homeopathic treatment of chronic conditions can bring you new health and happiness while adding a decade to your lifespan.

- Where to get help from skilled professional homeopaths who can cure—not just relieve—chronic allergies, arthritis, asthma, gout, heart disease, hypertension, depression, schizophrenia and most other psychological afflictions, hereditary disorders, infectious diseases, skin problems, major injuries, and deep chronic afflictions of every kind—even early stage cancer, multiple sclerosis and AIDS.

Safe home care for minor ailments:

- How the author's wife quickly learned to safely, swiftly cheaply treat her family and friends, joining the legion of homeopathic home prescribers across America. More than a dozen cured cases are presented.

- How to get yourself an inexpensive home treatment kit and books so you can safely, cheaply treat yourself and your family in the privacy and comfort of your home.

- What you can cure at home: anxiety, athlete's foot, backache, bites, bleeding, blisters, boils, bruises, burns, childhood illnesses,

by the end of this book, you'll know ...

choking, colds, constipation, cuts, dental pain, diarrhea, earaches, fainting, flus, gas, headaches, hemorroids, herpes simplex, impetigo, indigestion, jockitch, menopausal problems, minor injuries, motion sickness, nausea, overexertion, PMS, poison oak, pregnancy problems, rashes, ringworm, shingles, shin splints, shock, sore muscles, sore throat, sprains, stings, strains, styes, sunburn, vomiting, yeast infections ... and more.

- Where to get safe, non-toxic, cheap, FDA-approved non-prescription homeopathic remedies.

And...

- What homepathy can do for animals, infants and the aged and dying.

- What homeopathic physicians are like, from profiles of ten dedicated doctors.

- The dangers of routine vaccination—and how to avoid it.

- How to measure your own personal condition with the homeopathic Definition of Health.

- The discovery, history, philosophy, research, theory and pharmacy of this unique, wonderfully curative, sophisticated and scientific system of medicine.

Armed with all this knowledge you can wisely then decide what this proven, safe, holistic medicine can do for you. . . .

Other books by Robert S. Wood:

Desolation Wilderness	Good-Bye, Loneliness!
Pleasure Packing	The 2 Oz. Backpacker
Mountain Cabin	Whitewater Boatman

HOMEOPATHY
MEDICINE THAT
WORKS!

ROBERT S. WOOD

Condor Books
Pollock Pines, California

HOMEOPATHY: MEDICINE THAT WORKS!

Published by
Condor Books
2260 Forebay Road
Pollock Pines, California
95726

Distributed by
Publishers Services
P.O. Box 2510
Novato, California
94948

Cover and book design by Paula Morrison
Typeset by Campaigne & Associates Typography
Printed in the United States of America

Library of Congress Cataloging-in-Publication Data

Wood, Robert S., 1931–
    Homeopathy: medicine that works! / by Robert S. Wood.
        p.   cm.
    Includes bibliographical references (p.   )
    ISBN 0–913238–04–X
    1. Homeopathy.   I. Title.
RX71.W66   1990
615.5'32—dc20   90–45190
                                                       CIP

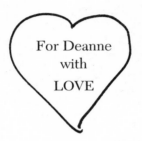

For Deanne
with
LOVE

Table of Contents

Acknowledgements

Thanks go first to my doctor, Bill Gray, who made my cure and this book possible. Next comes ever-dependable Hahnemann Pharmacist Michael Quinn, followed by Hawaii Naturopath Michael Traub.

My dear wife Deanne kept me happy and healthy throughout this project and was always there when I needed her.

I'm grateful to Richard Moskowitz for providing most of chapter 14, "The Case Against Vaccination," and to homeopathic veterinarian Richard H. Pitcairn for much of chapter 12, "Kids & Dogs Don't Lie!"

I'm obliged to George Vithoulkas and Grove Press for kind permission to present a condensation of the first section of *The Science of Homeopathy* in chapter 2, "How Homeopathy Works." And to Harris Coulter and George Vithoulkas for their contributions to chapter 1.

Richard Grossinger and Dana Ullman provided valuable criticism and editorial advice. Hahnemann Clinic homeopaths Roger Morrison, Peggy Chipkin, Matt Vuksinich, Vicky Menear, Jonathan Shore and Nancy Herrick all contributed variously to this book. So did Linda Johnston, Mark Allen and Ken Kehoe who introduced me to homeopathy.

And I'm indebted to the people who shared their personal cases ... and to the many who encouraged me when the publishing establishment rejected my work.

Finally, I want to thank the production team of designer Paula Morrison and typographer Campaigne & Associates for admirably transforming my manuscript into this book.

Bob Wood
Pollock Pines
Summer, 1990

Foreword

I probably shouldn't be introducing this book because I'm such a prominent part of it. But I'd like to say a few words from the viewpoint of a homeopathic doctor. This book is a gateway for the explorer into the strange but wonderfully curative world of homeopathy—a safe, inexpensive, sophisticated and scientific system of medicine now finally gaining the acceptance it deserves.

Most texts on the subject read like the telephone book. Now finally there's a fast-paced, accurate, exciting book that truly entertains while conveying the full depth and breadth of homeopathy—from acute ailments to deep chronic disease—in children and pets as well as adults. It's easily the best writing I've ever seen on the subject.

Right from the start you get involved with Bob's personal odyssey, his true-life adventure. He sucks you into the struggles, uncertainties, paradoxes and agonizing setbacks of his chronic allergy case. Once his story is underway, he jumps to the technical aspects of homeopathy.

After that, chapters on his case alternate with technical chapters on discovery, history, theory, philosophy, pharmacy, immunizations, veterinary, dentistry, curable chronic diseases and profiles of homeopaths. He finishes with a blaze of what we readers like best . . . the satisfying outcome of his case and many others.

Along the way the book is full of great success stories. In cases of all kinds we see homeopathy at work dramatically curing every sort of affliction from bee-stings to deeply seated chronic conditions. Like a fly on the wall you sit in my office and watch the drama unfold. You see the author's wife develop into an excellent homeopathic home prescriber, and watch the world master unravel a difficult case.

Bob has mustered considerable writing ability—and not a little personal courage—to open the way for others. The story of his growth is fascinating. Homeopathy produces a radical change in one's world-view regarding symptoms, medicines and cure. Bob has made that adventurous transition and willingly shares his experience.

He has opened the door to new possibilities, making it clear what homeopathy can do, what it costs, why it is becoming so popular, its drawbacks, the hope it offers to sufferers of all kinds. The book will be invaluable for people in search of curative treatment.

Bill Gray, M.D.
Hahnemann Medical Clinic

Introduction

What Is Homeopathy?

Hahnemann's Exciting Discovery . . . Basic Principles . . .
The News Spreads Worldwide . . . Dark Ages in America . . .
Homeopathy Rediscovered . . . Today's Boom . . . What
Homeopathy Can Cure

You might ask your grandmother. She may well remember those distant years when homeopathy (ho-me-AH-pa-thee) first flourished in America as a respected branch of medicine, with a cure rate beyond compare.

If your grandmother is like mine, she probably had a wooden rack of tiny vials of medicine with which she effectively and inexpensively treated her family. And if she *really* got sick, she went to a homeopathic physician, who painstakingly elicited the full range of her symptoms before prescribing a single remedy that couldn't possibly harm her.

It may seem hard to believe, but at the turn of the century, one out of every five doctors in America was a fully-licensed practicing homeopath. In the year 1900 there were 22 homeopathic medical schools, more than 100 homeopathic hospitals, 60 homes for orphans and the aged, over 1000 homeopathic pharmacies and 29 different homeopathic journals. Homeopathy was supported by such literary giants as Longfellow, Hawthorne and William James, endorsed by statesmen like Daniel Webster and Horace Greely, and magnate John D. Rockefeller.

So, what happened?

Homeopathy became a victim—temporarily—of its powerful, rich and determined competitor, the American medical establishment. But before returning to homeopathy's survival and resurgence, let's go back to the origins of what has been called, "the most effective system of medicine known to man."

The heart of homeopathy, the Law of Similars, goes back to the Hindu sages of the tenth century B.C. The Law appears in the writings of Hippocrates in 400 B.C. and it surfaces again in the words of the fifteenth century German physician Paracelus. The principle was utilized by the Mayans, Greeks, Chinese and American Indians. But it took the German genius Samuel Hahnemann to develop the principle into a systematic medical science in the late 1700's.

Hahnemann, an eminent physician and chemist who could read and write seven languages by the age of 24, gave up medicine in disgust because the treatments of the day were so barbarous and pitifully ineffective. Patients routinely were purged, blistered, cauterized and bled, while being heavily dosed with such poisons as arsenic and mercury. Only the strongest constitutions survived these heroic treatments!

Hahnemann was translating a medical textbook by one William Cullen, when he came across an explanation that so outraged his reason and medical knowledge that he decided to conclusively prove it wrong.

Cullen blithely attributed the effectiveness of Peruvian Bark (quinine) in treating malaria solely to its astringent bitterness. Hahnemann knew of many substances more astringently bitter— and none of them cured malaria. Curious now about Peruvian Bark's properties, he decided to take the herb himself. When repeated doses brought his healthy body to the point of toxicity, he developed, to his surprise, all the symptoms peculiar to malaria—fever and chills, anxiety and trembling.

Mere coincidence seemed unlikely. Hahnemann was familiar with the writings of Hippocrates and Paracelsus, so he had previously been exposed to the Law of Similars as theory. Now he had first hand evidence of its veracity. Peruvian Bark he deduced, cured malaria symptoms simply *because* it produced those exact same symptoms in a healthy person. He had discovered a fundamental law of cure and the first principle of homeopathy.

Excited by his discovery, he sought confirmation in the other common medicines of the day. Time after time he dosed himself with a drug to the point of toxicity, then scrupulously recorded his symptoms in great detail. Acting on his discovery, he then chose medicines for patients by matching their symptoms to the medicines that produced them.

Sure enough, the medicines were highly curative when matched to the patient solely on the basis of symptoms. And they worked holistically on the whole organism, curing mental and emotional afflictions as well as physical maladies. He had re-discovered and put to work The Law of Similars. He named his new medicine homeopathy: "homeo" meaning similar and "pathos" meaning suffering. Its guiding principle was, "Like cures like."

An exhaustive study by Hahnemann of poisonings in the medical literature of the time provided further confirmation. Toxic overdoses, it turned out, *always* produced the symptoms of the illnesses they could cure. Hahnemann's great discovery attracted a number of fellow physicians who were likewise searching for the means to truly cure. For the next six years the group systematically tested drugs, keeping meticulous records. These tests, made solely on healthy human beings, were called "provings."

When proven remedies were used according to Hahnemann's principle to treat the very symptoms they produced, all sorts of previously "incurable" cases were quickly and permanently cured, sometimes with only a single dose! To the medical world it was magic!

Hahnemann's second great discovery was "potentization." His remedies, though curative, were often toxic if taken too often, producing unwanted though temporary side effects. Diluting the medicine reduced the toxicity and side effects, but unfortunately it also reduced the medicine's effectiveness. Then he somehow discovered that vigorous shaking during each dilution actually *increased* the medicine's potency while decreasing toxicity! Modest

3

homeopaths don't pretend to know how the discovery took place or why it happens, but undeniably it works. It's been happening consistently for nearly 200 years!

This vigorous energizing during dilution Hahnemann called potentization. It proved to be a breakthrough. Utilizing this principle, he could minimize toxicity and at the same time increase a medicine's potency. The problem of side effects disappeared as the medicine became more potent.

Potentization is unquestionably the most controversial aspect of homeopathy because it seems to contradict our basic beliefs about dilution. As children we learned that dilution means weaker, but the addition of vigorous shaking actually reverses the process. In homeopathy, less turns out to be more. Potentization has been proven by 200 years of consistent clinical experience. It has also been scientifically validated by independent modern laboratory research. There's still a great deal we don't know about the human organism. In order to heal it, we sometimes must rely on empirical evidence. That's what homeopathy does.

It was clear to Hahnemann that since his remedies were too dilute to affect the tissues of his patients, their curative power must come from their ability to unleash the body's own impressive healing powers. When the remedy matched the patient's symptoms precisely, a kind of resonance occurred that somehow supercharged the body's own healing energy. This life energy he called the "vital force."

Before he was through, Hahnemann also proved the inseparability of body, mind and emotions. Proper diagnosis, it could be seen, required evaluating mental and emotional symptoms as well as the physical. And homeopathic cures took place on all three aspects of the organism. To complete his system, Hahnemann insisted on prescribing the smallest possible dose of the single remedy that best fit the totality of the patient's symptoms.

Symptoms, he came to realize, were merely positive adaptive responses of the body to all kinds of internal and external stress. They demonstrated the body's best efforts to heal itself. "Obliterating symptoms," it has been said, "is like killing the messenger for bringing bad news!" But obliterating symptoms is largely the basis for conventional medicine.

Hahnemann deduced that germs could not be the "cause" of disease. Germs by the millions live harmlessly in all of us. The cause of illness, he realized, was the pre-existing susceptibility or weakness of the individual. It was therefore necessary to treat the weakness, not the germ. And that's what homeopathic remedies do. Instead of working directly on germs, they work to strengthen the body's weakness. By contrast, antibiotics may destroy germs, but they weaken the body's defenses and have no effect whatever on the real causes of infection.

Before he died in 1843, at the age of 88, Hahnemann had personally conducted or supervised provings of 99 different substances. And he left behind a systematic, integrated, coherent, system of medicine with a cure rate unparalleled in history.

Its remedies were natural: single substances found in nature (animal, mineral or vegetable). They worked naturally to help heal the body, mind and emotions. When properly prescribed to fit the patient's own symptom picture, they strengthened the vital force sufficiently to effect lasting cures, instead of harshly drugging the body to suppress unwanted individual symptoms. By the year 1900 there were close to 700 proven remedies in the homeopath's arsenal.

Right from the start, homeopathy was scorned by the medical establishment, but popular with the grateful multitudes it cured. Homeopathy threatened conventional medicine in various ways: because its remedies were cheap it competed too effectively; it's principles ran contrary to established beliefs; it outperformed orthodox treatment; its medicines were different, dilute, and non-toxic . . . and homeopaths, led by Hahnemann, were sharply critical of the barbarities and failures of the medical establishment.

Nevertheless, homeopathy spread rapidly throughout Europe —because it worked! It found its way to America after its sensational success in treating victims of the terrible cholera epidemic of 1832 in Europe. The survival rate of those treated homeopathically was three times that of orthodox medicine! Since medical practices in America were also barbaric, and epidemics were common, the country was ripe for a safe, humane, effective system of cure.

Yellow fever, cholera, typhoid and scarlet fever swept our young nation in the 1800's, and homeopathic treatment proved two to eight times as successful as conventional medicine in treating these deadly epidemics. Thanks to these successes, homeopathy spread across the country like wildfire, and in 1844 the first national medical society in the U.S. was founded: The American Institute of Homeopathy!

Two years later, largely in retaliation, the American Medical Association (AMA) was organized, in part, as its charter proclaims, "to stamp out the scourge of homeopathy." Nevertheless, throughout the rest of the century, homeopathy grew rapidly in popularity as word spread of its safe, cheap and effective cures. It had become so successful by 1900 that the AMA and the already rich and powerful drug industry became alarmed. Homeopathy was competing far too successfully, cutting deeply into industry profits! So war was declared by the medical establishment!

An all-out campaign was mounted to discredit, thwart and undermine homeopathy, using influence, money and political clout. Homeopaths, by nature, have always been more interested in healing than fighting. So they didn't band together or react defensively. Gradually the concerted, well-bankrolled efforts of the medical establishment (doctors and drug companies) began to prevail.

Homeopaths were expelled from medical societies and their medical schools were financially squeezed until, one by one, they had to close for lack of funds. Without schools, medical students were forced to accept conventional medicine. There no longer was any alternative. Homeopathy was effectively subverted and repressed by its stronger, more aggressive competitors.

By 1920, homeopathy had entered a dark age in America. A scattering of homeopaths valiantly continued to practice, helping one another and keeping the art alive, but they were persecuted by the medical establishment at every turn and there were no new students to replace them when they grew old.

Meanwhile, unhindered by rapacious big business, homeopathy continued to spread and flourish in the rest of the world. In

6

Europe, most people know and use homeopathy. There are inexpensive remedies available from homeopathic pharmacies on every street corner in France, Germany and Italy. In England the Royal Family has relied on homeopathy since 1830. A recent survey showed that visits to homeopaths by Britons are currently increasing by 39% yearly! The impressive growth in England is being matched in France, where more than 20,000 French pharmacies sell homeopathic medicines. Six medical schools offer degrees in homeopathy, which is taught in all French pharmacy schools.

Homeopathy is even more popular in Asia, especially in India. One hundred thousand homeopaths practice in India, thanks in part to the endorsement of Mahatma Ghandi. And 120 homeopathic medical schools graduate thousands of new doctors each year.

In Africa, Australia, Central and South America, New Zealand and even Russia, homeopathy is flourishing. In Brazil, for instance, ten homeopathic medical schools have produced more than 2000 physicians. And Argentina has another 2000 who regularly treat three million people. All over the world, homeopathy has been recognized as a safe, inexpensive, marvelously effective means of treating not only physical symptoms, but mental and emotional disturbances as well.

But Americans are not stupid, and they refuse to remain ignorant. In the early 1970's they began to revolt. They were tired of being told that they had to accept crippling, often deadly side effects from their "miracle" drugs. They were tired of trading one symptom for something worse, of being put in the hospital by "wonder" drugs, or hearing from their doctors that there was something wrong with *them* because they got sicker instead of better.

They were tired of paying vast sums for medical treatment that failed to cure. They began to sense that holistic (whole person) treatment made more sense than simply obliterating unwanted symptoms. They began to suspect that mental and emotional disturbances were tied inseparably to physical disabilities.

Americans were fast losing faith in modern medicine. They began to refuse risky drugs. They stood up and looked around for alternatives, and they rediscovered homeopathy—and other natural, non-abusive means of healing that the AMA and the drug industry had long been trying to suppress and discredit. When word leaked out that "drug-reactions" always stand in the top ten causes of hospitalization, they began to question the wisdom of entrusting the nation's health to the multi-billion dollar drug industry.

With the rediscovery of holism in the early seventies, homeopathy began a rapid comeback. Dissatisfied MD's and medical students went to Europe and Greece and India to study homeopathy. And they returned to America to practice and teach, banding together now to protect themselves from persecution. The number of homeopaths doubled from 1980 to 1982. And from the early 1970's to the mid 1980's, the number increased one thousand percent!

At this writing there are now well over a thousand homeopathic MD's, plus another thousand licensed health professionals (dentists, nurses, naturopaths, physicians' assistants, chiropractors, veterinarians, acupuncturists and psychologists) . . . all practicing homeopathy. And hundreds more are on the way. In addition, there are thousands of lay prescribers, with thousands more to come as housewives and mothers learn to self-prescribe safe homeopathic remedies for their family's common complaints.

Sales of homeopathic remedies in America increased over one thousand percent from the late 1970's to the early 1980's, revealing the general public's enthusiastic response. After half a century, the dark age of homeopathy is finally over and the light is fast growing brighter. The good news is spreading fast. The American renaissance of homeopathy has begun.

If all this sounds intriguing but distinctly strange, that's understandable. We've learned by bitter experience to be suspicious of any system—especially a medical system—that promises great benefits without any drawbacks. Never-ending false medical claims have taught us to be skeptical. But there is truly no lasting downside to homeopathy. While many common ailments can be quickly healed, chronic cures take time so patience is required. And the patient must be able to tolerate healing crises called aggravations and the return of old symptoms. He or she must also be willing to actively participate in the process. Constitutional (chronic) homeopathy requires motivation and self-discipline.

But aggravations are only temporary and cures are long lasting, with no side effects to sabotage health. Homeopathy's dilute remedies act to heal the patient's system by means of curative stimulation—if they match his or her symptoms. If they don't, no harm is done. That's why they're safe for everyone, even suffering infants. And they genuinely cure—not merely relieve symptoms. Since homeopathy works holistically, it's as curative on the mental and emotional planes as it is on the physical. It can confer unimaginable blessings!

The need for safe cures has never been greater. More than a quarter of the country's population is chronically sick. And allergy, cancer, heart disease and immune system deficiencies like AIDS are on the rise. The eminent homeopath, Bill Gray, MD, has written, "homeopathy holds the answer for the vast majority of chronic disease sufferers." Even if you're basically healthy there's no better investment in the rest of your life than expert constitutional treatment. It can prevent untold suffering and add a decade to your life.

Homeopathy also works effectively in treating infectious diseases, gynecological conditions, digestive problems, skin diseases, colds, influenza, earaches, sore throats, headaches, childhood illnesses, accidents and even psychological and hereditary disorders.

In the pages that follow you will learn how and why homeopathy works, what it can cure (from bruises and colds to allergies and AIDS), why it's growing so fast in popularity, what it costs, how long it takes, its drawbacks—everything you need to know to evaluate its effectiveness. As the story of my case—and many other cases—unfold in story form, you will discover what it's actually like to experience homeopathic treatment. Homeopathic theory and philosophy are presented in depth in the words of the world master, George Vithoulkas.

Watching my wife Deanne evolve into an adept home prescriber, you'll see how easy it is to get a book and a kit and effectively, safely, inexpensively treat yourself and your family. You'll see homeopathy's application to dentistry and veterinary, meet homeopaths of all kinds, from budding converts to the world master, and learn how they found their way to the field. You'll read story after story of cured cases, followed by listings of sources, books, kits, organizations, doctors and clinics.

Armed with all that knowledge you can then wisely consider the potential of homeopathy to alleviate suffering in yourself or your loved ones. It can change your life by bringing radiant good health—and the happiness and freedom that real health makes possible.

Then, like Mark Twain, ". . . you may honestly feel grateful that homeopathy survived the attempts of the allopaths to destroy it."

1

Discovery & Diagnosis

My Chronic Hayfever Allergy . . . Constitutional
Homeopathic Treatment . . . The Hazards of Antidoting . . .
First Symptoms Appear . . . Two Revealing Books . . . My
First Follow-Up Visit . . . Aggravations Begin

I first heard of the wonders of homeopathy while sleepily soaking in a Death Valley swimming pool. It was Easter and the temperature hovered close to a hundred. The young man standing beside me happened to mention that he'd been cured by homeopathy of a debilitating pollen allergy that sounded very much like mine. That woke me up.

My chronic fall hay fever was always on my mind. For years I'd been searching for a cure without success. I told Ken my story. My wife and daughter and I lived on a wild river in the high desert just east of the California High Sierra near Lake Tahoe. I wrote health and outdoor books, several of them bestsellers, and Deanne taught high school. It was a wonderful place to live—except that I was deathly allergic to the ocean of rabbit brush and sage that blossomed every year from August to November. When the desert was in bloom I had to leave home. I simply couldn't stand it, no matter what medicine I tried. My problem was so severe that we were talking about selling our beloved home on the river.

Ken listened to my story, then he told me his. He'd lived on a farm where they raised alfalfa, and he'd been miserable from the moment it came into bloom. He'd taken his problem to an old German homeopath in San Francisco, who'd given him a tiny bottle of pills to take. "The first year," he told me, "I wasn't much better. The second year I didn't sneeze half as much. The third year I had hardly any trouble at all. And the problem never came back. I was cured."

I prodded for more information but all I learned was that homeopathy worked on the whole body and was safe and cheap, with no side effects. He didn't remember the name of his doctor but there was supposed to be an excellent homeopathic clinic in Berkeley. He couldn't remember its name either, but it sounded like some kind of fish . . . maybe mackerel . . . or haddock.

As soon as we got back to our home in the desert we started hunting. The fall allergy season was now only five months away. In our five-year-old Berkeley phone book we found a "Hering Family Clinic." When I called the operator told me that Hering was out of business, and the number now belonged to Hahnemann Family Clinic. It seemed a longshot but I called.

A lady named Karen with an English accent assured me I had the right place: Hering had recently been reorganized into Hahnemann and was the only homeopathic clinic in the area. Looking in that old phone book had been a piece of luck because a new one wouldn't have shown Hering. Apparently I was meant to make contact.

When Karen suggested I drop in and talk to a doctor, I told her I lived 250 miles away over the mountains. She gave me the phone number of the International Foundation for Homeopathy in Seattle and said they might know of a clinic that was closer.

She was wrong. The lady on the telephone in Seattle told me Berkeley was the closest and probably the best of a handful of classical homeopathic clinics in America. She sympathized with the distance to be traveled but told me that frequent trips shouldn't be necessary. She introduced herself as Rosalyn and politely asked the nature of my problem. When I told her about my pollen allergy she strongly urged me to call Hahnemann back.

"Don't give up on them because of the distance," she urged. "They can cure your hay fever. I *know* they can. Homeopathy has

12

changed my life. And my daughter's, too." She wouldn't let me off the long distance line until I promised to call Hahnemann and get more information.

When I called Karen back she promised to have the doctor who had 'Phone Duty' that day call me collect. His name, she said, was Bill Gray. He was an MD and happened to be one of America's foremost homeopaths. When he called an hour later, he sounded both professional and frank. When he asked what I knew about homeopathy, I repeated what Ken and Rosalyn had told me, and I answered his questions about my allergy.

"I would say there's an 80–90% chance we can cure you completely," he said soberly. "But it would take three years. You wouldn't be much better the first pollen season, but you'd be more than 50% better the second. And the third year you ought to be nearly symptom free. I want to stress that I really mean *cure*, not just symptom relief. And our remedies are completely safe, without side effects or risk. All you have to supply is the patience."

He explained the procedure. First, came an interview in which the homeopath extensively questioned the patient in an effort to classify him precisely as an individual. It would take at least an hour. When the homeopath was confident of the remedy required, it would be supplied by the Clinic's own pharmacy. Then the remedy—usually in the form of treated sugar pills—would be swallowed. The first followup appointment would be 4–6 weeks later, to see if the remedy was working. Intensified allergy symptoms would indicate progress.

After that there would be occasional checkups, which in my case might be managed by phone, for several years.

"I'd only have to make the trip twice?"

"Right . . . providing the first remedy works."

I was ready. There seemed so much to gain and nothing to lose. I said I'd like to make the first appointment for the following week when we'd be at our summer cabin in the mountains, a hundred miles closer to Berkeley.

Like the Indians before us, my wife and daughter and I migrate from the warming desert every spring to spend the summer in the cool high Sierra at our rustic cabin on Echo Lake. We had hardly settled in before it was time for my appointment with Dr. Gray in Berkeley.

Going back to Berkeley was going home. Like my mother before me, I had been born in the University town by San Francisco Bay and I had lived there for half a century, writing for *Life* and *Time* magazines, before saying goodbye to life in the city. My mother still lived in the house where I grew up. When I told her I was about to try homeopathic treatment for my pollen allergy, she said, "That's certainly appropriate. Your great grandmother treated herself and her family from a wooden rack of little bottles of homeopathic remedies. So did your grandmother."

Hahnemann Clinic turned out to be a handsome, two-story colonial brick building. When I stepped through the door I found myself in a classic Greek temple. Simulated marble walls rose from a flagstone terrace to a ceiling of clouds. Square marble columns around the room's perimeter each bore a gold plaque on which was inscribed a homeopathic remedy. Light shown down from a ragged recess in the ceiling, as though from a rent in storm clouds. Delightful!

I made my way to a counter-height opening in one marble wall where Karen sat at a reception desk. She welcomed me, gave me several forms and directed me to a staircase. Upstairs, I found a conventional doctor's waiting room. I was immediately ushered into a small examination cubicle where a nurse took my temperature, pulse and blood pressure, weighed me, asked if I was taking any medicine or drugs (I wasn't) and entered this information on one of my forms.

Then I sat down to wait for Dr. Gray. I was looking forward to the homeopathic interview. What could be more fun than talking about myself and my background? As I waited, I mentally reviewed my health history.

All through my youth I had been sickly and allergic. It wasn't until college that I finally outgrew my asthma and most of my food allergies. But the problems that remained required me to take allergy shots every three weeks. And low grade symptoms were more or less continuous: especially hayfever and nasal blockage that prevented me from breathing through my nose. I carried a squeeze bottle of antihistamine nose drops in my pocket, taking a sniff every few hours to temporarily clear my nostrils.

By my early thirties I had finally grown disgusted with the pitiful offerings of allopathic (conventional) medicine. My allergist made it clear that he expected me to take his allergy shots for the rest of my life. It would be far too risky, he said, to quit.

Dissatisfied with this prescription, I looked around for something better. A friend pointed me to a chiropractic internist who had helped a lot of people who had been sentenced by allopaths to a lifetime of ineffectual drugs. Like them I was willing to try something new.

Within a month Dr. William Nelson, D.C., in San Francisco, had dispatched my chronic lower back pain and tennis elbow. And after two months, holding my breath, I skipped my allergy shot for the first time in ten years—without the slightest consequence! (I never went back for another.) After the third month of treatment I had also broken my addiction to the nose drops which were gradually destroying the lining of my nose. I went to see Dr. Nelson for many years but my allergies never got much better. I never knew what it meant to breathe through my nose like everybody else.

In my early forties I came to wonder why I wasn't happier despite modest success in various fields. My real estate investments had allowed me to retire at the age of 34 from my position as *Life* Correspondent in San Francisco, and I had written half a dozen books. I lived in a beautiful Berkeley home with my first wife and daughter and spent a quarter of the year at my cabin in the mountains. I had everything I wanted, but I wasn't really happy.

Then one day a friend brought me a book that so excited and disturbed her that she couldn't sleep. She insisted my wife and I read it *immediately* and tell her what we thought. It was Arthur Janov's *The Primal Scream,* and we found it so compelling that within a month we were all in primal therapy. The journal I kept of my experiences became a book entitled *Goodbye, Loneliness!* (Dell, 1974). In it I detailed the tranformation (part emotional, part mental and physical) that brought me a peace and contentment I had never known before. Primal has its hazards and the cure rate is low, but it worked wonderfully for me.

In the past ten years I had integrated the gains I made in therapy, and I had found two more men with magic in their hands who called themselves chiropractors. Eight years before, a surgeon had operated on my nose to give me normal sized passages, but the linings remained swollen by low grade allergies. When my first wife and I divorced I moved to the house in the desert and its sea of malignant sage. Within two years I had remarried—and developed my devastating allergy.

Twenty minutes had passed since I sat down in the waiting room and I began to wonder if I'd been forgotten. Finally, a pleasant looking man of average height and stocky build, aged perhaps 45, came into the waiting room and spoke my name in a soft tenor voice. He was wearing grey slacks, a white shirt, a conservative tie . . . and no white coat. He introduced himself simply as Bill Gray. Then he led me to a large windowless office where I sat down in a chair in front of his desk.

He leaned back in his oak swivel chair with his hands behind his head and asked about some outdoor books I had written. I wondered when the searching interview would begin. His manner was so easy and natural that it never occurred to me that he had been sizing me up since the moment he first saw me and had already made several important judgements. I didn't know then that a good homeopath, besides knowing the symptomology of some 800 remedies, must also be a skilled psychologist and shrewd detective.

As he sipped from a mug of tea he asked what sounded like casual questions about my medical history. I told him as concisely as I could about my early allergies, the shots I had taken and my nose operation. I went into more detail, at his urging, about Dr. Nelson's treatments and the transformation that resulted from primal therapy.

The interview moved briskly. He fired questions and I tried to provide succinct answers. He rarely had to interrupt, yet he changed the subject often with deftness and speed. After perhaps twenty minutes he began to scribble rapidly on a sheet of paper,

16

and he occasionally leafed through one of several huge, dog-eared, leather-bound black reference books on his desk. When he found what he wanted, he made a hasty note then framed a new question. When a page was full he set it to one side and snatched another.

As the pages began to pile up, Dr. Gray seemed to slow down. I got the feeling that he was exploring one blind alley after another. After another twenty minutes he seemed to be stymied. He leaned back in his chair and stared at the ceiling for several minutes, then he re-read his notes. (By now there were five pages.) Then it was back to his medical encyclopedias. He frowned and gazed again at the ceiling. I silently urged him to keep trying. Together we could surely find the answer.

For the past twenty minutes he had been asking me about my reactions to heat and cold, my sensitivity to changes in the weather and details of my sleep habits. It seemed to make a big difference that I slept best on my left side, never on my back or stomach and was inclined to heartburn if I slept on my right side for very long.

Although he had been extremely attentive as I explained my passage through primal therapy, he now asked precise questions about my mental and emotional state, especially about anxieties, moods and depressions. When I told him I was one of the least fearful people I knew, he turned to my eating habits. I told him I rarely ate breakfast because I simply wasn't hungry first thing in the morning. When he asked what foods I craved most, I said I hadn't any cravings. He wasn't satisfied. "Well then what would you say are your favorite foods?"

"Well, I like butter and bacon and. . . ."

"Did you say bacon?"

"Yes. I love bacon . . . fried crisp."

He flipped through a thick black book. When he found what he wanted he asked, "Anybody in your family ever had tuberculosis?"

"Yes, my dad had TB as a teenager."

"Good," he said briskly. "How do you feel about cats?"

"I don't care for cats. Cat dander used to give me asthma as a kid. Cats always seek me out, though. Somehow they know I don't like them."

He nodded and turned back to his reference books. He read for quite awhile before leaning back in his chair, eyeing me speculatively. Then, with a trace of a smile, he asked, "This may sound funny, but how do you feel about pine trees?"

"I love them!" I burst out. I'd never thought about it before, but it was undeniably true. I told him I'd even majored in forestry in college!

Before I could amplify he leaned forward to ask, "How much of that is esthetic?"

I stopped to think. "Well, there is certainly an esthetic element," I admitted, "but I'm genuinely fond of them apart from all that. I've always had the best associations with pine trees." I hesitated. "In fact, I've even been known to hug them! I like the smell of the pitch, especially of Jeffery and Pinon Pine and. . . ."

He sat back smiling, letting me babble on. It was clear he'd struck oil. "We've got a pretty good picture now with your craving for bacon, the affinity for pine trees, your aversion to cats and your dad's TB. It all points to Tuberculinum. So that's what I'm going to give you. I think it will work."

"As in . . . tuberculosis?"

He nodded. "Tuberculinum is made from tissue from a tubercular cow. If it works you'll be getting a return of your most recent allergic symptoms. But that's a good sign. Don't treat your symptoms in any way. Understand? No medicines of any kind. Okay?"

He waited for my assent before continuing. "Overall, you're in pretty good shape . . . thanks mainly to the primal therapy and chiropractic work. They probably cleared up a lot of your mental and emotional symptoms . . . as well as the congestion in your chest."

He went on to tell me there were a few things I must avoid because they could "antidote" any homeopathic remedy. Coffee beans and camphor were strictly forbidden. I showed him the tube of Mentholatum Lip Balm I always carried in my pocket for dry lips. He read the ingredients, smelled it and handed it back. "It doesn't list camphor so I think it's all right."

To show I had done my homework, I asked, "What about dental work? The flyer said to postpone routine dental work for three years. I assume that's a typo," I chuckled. "Did you mean three weeks or three days?"

"We mean three years," he said seriously. "Dental drilling seems to cause a resonance in the bone that can antidote remedies, stopping the work of the vital force. But routine cleaning is okay."

He watched me to see how this news was received. "Do you have a lot of problems with your teeth?"

I felt a trifle foolish. "No, but three years is a long time. What if I'm in pain and really need something done?"

"Call me first and I'll advise you. If you're in pain, you'll probably need dental work. If the drilling stops the process we'll do our best to get it going again."

I slowly nodded. No cavities for three years? It was a sobering thought. I'd been averaging at least one a year.

"I'll want to see you again in four weeks," he told me. "Try to be aware of any changes in your symptoms during that time, so you can tell me what happened, especially during the first few days."

"I'll keep a journal," I offered.

He nodded. "I won't need that much detail, at least not day by day, but write things down as they happen . . . so you don't forget."

He handed me a prescription, and I asked if he would recommend a couple of books on homeopathy. He said there was a blue one for sale in the waiting room that would introduce me to the subject. It was by George Vithoulkas, the Greek homeopath with whom he had studied, the leading practitioner alive. I thanked him and went to the pharmacy. The proprietor, a tall earnest young man named Michael Quinn, took my prescription and disappeared. After several minutes he returned with a tiny vial the diameter of a pencil and barely an inch long.

"Here's your remedy," he said. "If you haven't eaten recently, you can take the full contents right now."

I opened the vial. Inside were tiny white pellets.

"They're sugar pills," he explained. "The remedy is a very dilute coating on the outside."

I asked what he thought about my Mentholatum Lip Balm.

He carefully read the ingredients and smelled it. "I'm pretty conservative so I wouldn't take it," he advised.

When I told him I had to have something for the dry mountain air that cracked my lips, he suggested plain Chapstick, "the black one without any flavor or smell." I said I had some at home.

When I asked him to recommend reading material, he took me to a bookcase containing more than a dozen different titles. He picked them up one by one and gave me a brief review of each, highly recommending the blue book Dr. Gray had mentioned, *Homeopathy: Medicine of the New Man* by George Vithoulkas. I didn't know then that the book had been ghost-written by my doctor while he was studying in Greece.

I also bought *Homeopathic Medicine,* a little orange book by Harris L. Coulter, that Michael said represented a very different point of view of homeopathy. The bill for the two books—plus my remedy—was $13.21.

"Are you going to take the remedy now?" Michael gently reminded me.

"Sure. Why not?" I tipped back my head, poured the pills in my mouth, chewed a couple of times and swallowed. Then I had a sobering thought. I could no longer use camphor or drink coffee. It would be years before I could have my teeth drilled. I felt a twinge of anxiety, but it quickly passed. I felt elated as I paid my bill for the hour's interview and stepped out of the Greek temple to the tree-shaded street. I was on my way, with a fresh chance to escape the allergies that had plagued me all my life . . . and kept me from breathing through my nose.

That night, after driving back to our summer cabin in the mountains, I immediately received my first test. Deanne had wrenched a shoulder and was waiting impatiently for me to rub Ben Gay on her back. She took the cap off the tube and thrust it toward me. I could smell the distinctive aroma. I took it but something made me hesitate.

"Come on," she said, "our guests will be arriving any minute!"

"Does this have camphor in it?" I asked.

She quickly read the list of ingredients. "Yes, what about it?"

20

I handed back the tube. "I'm sorry, I'm not allowed to touch camphor."

I felt a little shaky. I'd come so close to antidoting my remedy the very first chance I got! On my way out to the bonfire with our neighbors, I grabbed one of the old black Chapstick tubes that Michael was sure would be okay. My lips were dry and I gratefully smeared on the soothing salve. During the course of the evening I applied some more. When our company had gone home, I recounted my day in detail by the dying campfire, ending with my use of the black Chapstick.

"Let me see that!" Deanne demanded.

I handed it over.

She turned on a flashlight to read the list of ingredients. "I thought so!" she cried. "It's got camphor in it!"

"Oh, no!" I felt sweat break out on my scalp. After barely escaping the Ben Gay, I had fallen prey to the Chapstick! How ironic that I'd traded my probably harmless Mentholatum for something that contained camphor! I'd scarcely been aware of camphor before. Now it seemed to be everywhere, threatening to antidote the remedy I'd driven so far to find. I felt stupid and miserable. There was nothing to do now but hope the dosage I'd received was insufficient to destroy the Tuberculinum.

Since there was no way for me to tell, I decided to postpone calling Dr. Gray until after the weekend. Hopefully, by then, I'd have symptoms to report. They weren't long in coming. Within twenty-four hours I wrote in my journal, "Periods of acute itching, corner of left eye and forehead." These, I remembered, were my most recent allergy symptoms . . . a good sign. Maybe I hadn't blown it with the camphor after all!

By Monday morning my journal also contained references to episodes of unexpected sinus and nasal congestion and an inability to sleep during afternoon naps. Wonderful!

When I called the clinic on Monday Karen told me Dr. Gray was busy with a patient but Michael could probably help me. When I candidly told the pharmacist about using the unflavored Chapstick, he quickly asked, "Was it old?"

"Yes, it even had a metal tube."

"That's old, all right. Did it smell?"

"Not that I remember."

"Good. You're probably okay then. Camphor vaporizes fairly quickly. If the Chapstick was old, most of the camphor had probably evaporated."

I felt relieved. Then I asked if my normal intake of three grams daily of vitamin C was okay. I had forgotten to tell Dr. Gray about that.

"Three grams gets to be medicinal," he warned. "I'd cut back to one."

Soon after returning, I began to read the blue book. At first I merely hoped to find out what I'd put in my body. And I was curious about the theory behind a method of treatment that could offer an 80–90% chance of cure in three years. In the Foreword, by my physician Bill Gray, I learned that as a young doctor he'd been bitterly disappointed by the failure of allopathic (orthodox) medicine to actually "cure." In search of something better, he had turned to holistic (whole body) healing.

One after another he'd studied nutrition, herbal medicine, acupuncture, chiropractic and polarity massage. But nothing he tried could consistently cure deep chronic disorders—until he discovered homeopathy. He was so impressed that he closed his practice in California and went to Greece to study with the world master, George Vithoulkas. There he learned how to provide his patients with precise, natural, non-toxic cures—the goal of conscientious physicians everywhere.

The text of the blue book began with history. I read how idealistic medical genius Samuel Hahnemann, in the early 1800's, stumbled onto a fundamental law, first stated by Hippocrates as "like cures like." Using himself as a guinea pig, he began to test the remedies of the day on himself, stubbornly, almost passionately persisting until he had devised a comprehensive and logical system of treatment with an unmatched record of cure.

Homeopathy, I learned, means "the treatment of suffering with a medicine that produces the identical kind of suffering."

Instead of using drugs to relieve symptoms like your orthodox doctor, the homeopath makes an exhaustive study of his patient's symptoms in order to find the pattern that corresponds exactly to the single homeopathic remedy that will produce that same pattern of symptoms in a normal healthy person. In my case, Tuberculinum. By matching the remedy pattern to the pattern of the patient, a powerful resonance is produced within the body. This mighty force will then annihilate the disturbance that is producing the symptoms, permitting the body to heal itself.

No one is quite sure exactly how it works, but undeniably it does. Two hundred years of consistent results prove that. A substance that produces certain symptoms in a healthy person will somehow cure those same symptoms in the person afflicted. And time has had no effect on what Hahnemann learned. Remedies that were effective two hundred years ago are just as healing today.

As I read I began to see an impeccable logic, a system based on reason and impressive results, an approach to disease and healing that was truly scientific and incredibly precise—never mind it's relative obscurity. I began to see why Vithoulkas claimed, "Only the person with . . . understanding and insight will choose homeopathy . . . only those who deserve it will find it and benefit." It was a thinking man's system, a reward for the true seeker.

It looked like I was on to something good, maybe great. But I didn't get really excited until I came to the last chapter, a brief 30-page Materia Medica that presented condensed symptom pictures of four common homeopathic remedies. These multi-dimensional portraits of remedy-conditions read like character sketches for a novel.

But what excited me most was that deep and complex mental and emotional afflictions could be cured, often quickly and dramatically, with such common non-toxic (and highly dilute) substances as Lycopodium (Club Moss) and Natrum muriaticum (common table salt)! It was hard to believe. Consider a few excerpts.

"Lycopodium patients are constantly contending with cowardice . . . (they) seek sexual gratification without the personal responsibilities implicit in such intimacy . . . (they) feel a deep sense of inadequacy and weakness . . . are in constant fear that others will discover their inner state of weakness . . . (so they) go overboard in presenting a bluff to compensate for inner feelings of inferiority.... "They exaggerate their attainments . . . tell outrageous lies . . . become dictatorial and tyrannical with those who can be controlled.... They can become terrified by almost anything—-being alone, the dark, ghosts, even straydogs . . . their fears and anxieties affect mostly the gastrointestinal tract . . . there is an emaciation of the face, neck and upper torso . . ." etc., etc.

And "Natrum muriaticum patients are emotionally very sensitive . . . but quite clear and strong on mental and physical levels.... They turn to introverted activities: reading books, listening to music.... Personal humiliation would be the end of the world for them . . . they become very serious . . . have a strong desire for salt and an aversion to slimy food, fat and chicken . . . an intolerance to heat, a sensitivity to light and both heat and cold. Moods swing from unreasonable depression to unreasonable exhilaration. A hypochondriacal anxiety about health emerges, a compulsive need to avoid contamination—always cleaning, washing hands, disinfecting everything.... Finally, they become shameless, exhibitionistic, speak in obscenities," etc.

Yet all these deep emotional and mental afflictions, the book asserted, could actually be cured with an incredibly dilute remedy made from simple salt! Unbelievable. (But don't try to diagnose on the basis of these brief glimpses. It's not nearly as easy as that!)

Michael the pharmacist had told me that the orange book, *Homeopathic Medicine* by Harris L. Coulter, took a different approach to the subject. And he was right. A medical historian, not a homeopath, Coulter seeks to put the precision, logic and reason I had found in homeopathy into sharp focus by comparing it in various respects to allopathic medicine. In doing so he makes a shambles of allopathy. In summary, he says. . . .

The allopath is superficially interested in the patient's general and most obvious symptoms in order to quickly place him in a broad disease category, so he can prescribe a broad-spectrum, devastatingly powerful and insufficiently tested drug, with the purpose of obliterating the offending symptoms—while producing new symptoms known as "side effects." He believes that disease entities are somehow separate from the symptoms exhibited, but that symptoms are always "harmful manifestations" of disease. The patient is expected to accept the new symptoms as the inevitable price of relief.

The homeopath, on the other hand, works his way quickly through the patient's general symptoms, then takes all the time necessary, during an exhaustive inquiry, to discover the subtle individual symptoms that reveal both the affliction and the single, utterly harmless remedy that exactly matches those symptoms . . . and therefore will effect a complete and lasting cure. To the homeopath, symptoms are entirely benign. They merely constitute the evidence of the efforts being made by the body's vital force to rid itself of the affliction. (The vital force may be defined as the mysterious inner intelligence in each of us that governs the organism and strives to maintain its health.)

The allopath operates under no explicit set of assumptions, no general theory, except that symptoms are bad, and roughly grouped together they constitute certain diseases, according to a vague pattern. He rejects holism (i.e. treatment of the entire organism) and the concept of the vital force. And he ignores individual susceptibility, preferring to prescribe solely on the basis of disease from an arsenal of 30–40 powerful drugs that produce a host of debilitating (and sometimes deadly) side effects.

He is overly proud of the precision of the exhaustive testing which he usually delegates to his subordinates—even though the highly refined data produced often has no therapeutic application.

The homeopath operates under an admirably systematized, thoroughly logical, precise theory of medicine. He administers a single, harmless, dilute remedy which is perfectly matched to the totality of the patient's symptoms. His stable and scientific approach, based on the fundamental Law of Similars, holistically cures and has been curing patients for 150 years. His arsenal contains more than 2000 remedies, of which he regularly prescribes some 300, and all of them are harmless and non-toxic.

While the homeopath enjoys a phenomenally high rate of cure without risk to the patient, the allopath suffers from unreliability, ambiguity and hopes only to relieve symptoms. As early as the mid-sixties, up to 40% of hospital admissions were for iatrogenic (drug-induced) illnesses, i.e. severe and sometimes fatal side effects from allopathic prescriptions. Cancer, arthritis, mental illness and heart disease are steadily increasing their toll as increasingly powerful drugs are used with less and less discrimination, as predicted decades ago by homeopathic physicians.

At present a third of the nation's hospital beds are filled with mental patients. Homeopathic theory shows that many of these illnesses were caused by powerful drugs used to massively suppress physical symptoms, thereby transferring the pathology to the brain! The rising incidence of chronic disease (e.g. allergies) doubtless shares the same origin. And many of the patients that allopaths claim to cure only enjoy a temporary suppression of symptoms. It may be months or years before the cures wear off and the same or other symptoms appear, or the patient finally reacts to the massive and improper medication.

In the next three weeks my symptoms slowly got worse. The itching on my forehead grew intense at times for no discernible reason. First it spread to my temples, then to my scalp, finally descending below my brow to my cheeks. Deanne removed all the lip preparations from my trouser pockets and the bathroom shelves as a precaution to prevent further "mistakes." I limited myself to coatings of Vaseline on my lips. Several times, absent-mindedly, I nearly accepted cups of decaffienated coffee from well-meaning friends, but I always caught myself in time—or Deanne declined for me.

Four weeks to the day from my first visit to the Clinic, I was back in Dr. Gray's office. The first thing I did was confess my indiscretion with the camphorated Chapstick. The doctor chuckled, agreeing with Michael that it hadn't done me any harm. He questioned me closely about my symptoms during the past four weeks, but made no effort to physically examine me. From where he sat he could easily see the redness between my eyebrows and at the corner of my left eye. He repeatedly asked about possible mental or emotional changes. I was steadfast in assuring him I'd detected none whatever. After ten minutes of intense questioning, he leaned back in his chair, arms behind his head.

"I'm 95% sure the remedy is working," he said at last. "The

dose I gave you should last another four to six months. Then I'll be giving you something different."

"We leave for Hawaii in four months and we plan to stay there about six months," I told him. "Can you give me the new prescription before we go?"

He nodded. "The timing should be just about perfect. I want to see you during the height of the sage pollen season, when your symptoms are at their worst. In the meantime we've got a small problem with your forehead inflammation. It should have stopped by now. Are you putting something on it?"

"Just Vaseline."

"How often?"

"At least six times a day."

"Hmmm. You better stop. I think it's prolonging the reaction."

"Stop using Vaseline?" I was aghast. I couldn't do without it. My skin would shrivel and dry to leather. "But isn't Vaseline inert?"

"I think it's aggravating your condition," he said firmly.

All at once I realized he was right. I had rubbed on Vaseline that morning, only half an hour before my appointment. My forehead hadn't been itching at the time, but now it was itching so infernally I couldn't keep from scratching for more than a minute—as he of course had noticed.

Even though the Vaseline apparently made me itch, I couldn't imagine being without it. I badly wanted to tell him how dry my skin had always been and how low the humidity was at both our desert and mountain homes. But he was right about the aggravation, so he must know what he was doing.

He seemed to read my mind. "You'll just have to tough it out, I'm afraid," he said gently. "I don't want you to put anything at all on your face, and that includes your lips."

Inwardly I groaned. My God! My lips, too? I'd carried some kind of salve for my lips in my pocket all my life. I couldn't go two hours without a fresh application!

"You're entering a critical period," he explained. "I don't want you to use anything that could mask or counteract your symptoms in any way. It might stop the process. If your skin gets too dry, eat more fat and oil . . . since you haven't a cholesterol problem."

I nodded. Oil sounded awful, but maybe I could live on butter and bacon.

"What else are you taking?" he wanted to know.

"Sometimes at night I need an antacid for heartburn if I've had spicy foods or sweets."

"No more antacid tablets."

I nodded, grimacing to myself. What was I supposed to do when the heartburn hit me in the night? How was I supposed to go back to sleep with a raging acid stomach? But I said nothing. Before I left he asked to me to call him in four weeks.

On the long drive back to the mountains I felt pleased that the remedy was working, but apprehensive about life without Vaseline, lip balm and Rolaids. It was going to be an experience! On the way I stopped to report to a friend. Jeannie had been using homeopathic remedies for years but had never been to a classical homeopath. After listening to my account she told me I was probably in for more aggravations, the increase in old symptoms that comes before the cure.

During the three hour journey my face gradually dried out as the last of the morning's Vaseline wore off. To my surprise I felt better instead of worse! The intense itching I had experienced at the Clinic was gone. I realized now that for weeks my itching face had been worse about an hour after rubbing on Vaseline!

Back at the cabin, Deanne demanded a detailed account of my visit. She didn't want a repetition of the Ben Gay and Chapstick fiascos. The next thing I knew, the various jars of Vaseline I had spotted around the cabin had vanished, the Rolaids were gone from the bedstand and bathroom, and my trouser pockets had been emptied of Chapstick. She didn't believe in fooling around— or leaving temptation in my path!

Jeannie's 'aggravations' began in earnest the next day. My face felt like parchment and my lips seemed to burn with every breath. I licked them incessantly, which of course made them worse. But my brow was no longer red and the maddening itch on my forehead was gone. Amazing!

In the days and weeks that followed my face and lips grew

steadily drier. My skin was tight and my face was chapped and constantly flaking, but I soon got used to it and wasn't really bothered. At first I used hot water and a wash cloth to remove the excess scale—until I discovered I was making my skin drier.

So, I stopped using soap and water on my face, hoping that the natural oils in my skin—long buried under Vaseline—would gradually return. And finally they did. By the third week I was no longer conscious of the dryness. When I took a shower now I took pains not to let my face get wet. If it did, I'd gently pat it dry, being careful not to remove the precious accumulation of natural oils.

At Dr. Gray's suggestion—and Deanne's urging—I increased the fat in my diet in hopes of making my flaky skin oilier. When we had steak, everyone passed me their fat. I didn't stint on butter. And Deanne served my beloved bacon with waffles for breakfast, in BLTs and hamburgers at lunch, and with liver and onions for dinner. In time my face became oilier—as much from my refusal to wash as from the extra fat I consumed.

Giving up Rolaids at night was murder—at first. I would wake with searing heartburn and sleepily reach for the jar that spelled relief. But it wasn't there any more. Deanne had seen to that! All I could do was take a sip of water from the glass on the bedstand, roll over on my left side—and hope. Usually the burning would gradually subside and permit me to go back to sleep. I soon learned not to sleep on my right side—ever!

In the second week a red welt appeared on the left side of my crotch. It might have been the return of the jock itch that had deviled me off and on since college days, but somehow it looked different. I hoped it was a sign that the Tuberculinum was working. A downward progression of symptoms was supposed to be good. A few days later I developed a crust on my left eyelid and the left side of my nose.

In the third week I was cheered by an itchy blistering between my fourth and baby toe, also on the left side. It didn't seem likely that this was a recurrence of athlete's foot because the climate was so dry and I was nearly always barefoot. I put nothing on any of these eruptions—mainly because I'd been told not to. But I was also afraid that they might go away, proving that they weren't the work of the Tuberculinum after all! I occasionally practiced introspection, too, hoping to detect mental or emotional changes.

I wish I could say I never cheated on Dr Gray's strictures. One night in the third week, after a day in the water, the skin on my brow felt like the head of a drum and looked like hamburger. A big flake of skin had come off, leaving a pink spot. Deanne happened to be administering Neosporin to a cut on her leg at the time.

"You poor thing," she sympathized. "Let me put a drop of this on your sore."

I did nothing to stop her. The next day it looked and felt much better, but I felt guilty and I couldn't help wondering if I'd hurt my chance of a cure. And I have to confess that I occasionally put the tiniest smidgen of Vaseline on my lips when they were burning from salt or too much licking—or the continual drying that comes from breathing almost exclusively through one's mouth. My fall from grace began when I discovered the sweet relief that came from kissing Deanne right after she had anointed her lips with Mentholatum Lip Balm—camphor-free, of course.

One day, after enviously watching her coat her lips, instead of kissing her I grabbed the Lip Balm, cried, "Enough of this subterfuge!" and rubbed a skimpy coating on my mouth. After that, I occasionally coated my lips if they were bothering me. In between times I kissed my pretty bride a lot! After all, before I could get well I had to survive! I would deal with the consequences later. There was still a full week before time to call Dr. Gray and report.

2

How Homeopathy Works

Humanity Defined ... The Three Dynamic Planes ...
Mental Aberrations ... The Measure of Health ... The Vital
Force ... The Defense Mechanism ... Homeopathic
Resonance ... Like Cures Like ... Potentization ... The
Major Threats ... The Worst Drugs ... Dangers of
Vaccination ... Hereditary Susceptibility.

The Greek master, George Vithoulkas, author of the "blue book,"
has written the definitive textbook on homeopathy. Called *The
Science of Homeopathy*, it has probably turned more pilgrims to
homeopathy—especially disenchanted allopaths—than any other
agency or event. So, there seems no better way to clearly and suc-
cinctly present the mysteriously appealing fundamentals of homeopathy than to condense the book's first section, "The Laws and
Principles of Cure."

George begins with the nature of the human organism and
works his way, step by step through the fundamentals of disease
and cure to the sublimely logical and effective theory of homeopathy, which he calls "the divine science."

The book's introduction points out that "orthodox medicine
is the only branch of science that has based its structure on opin-
ions and suppositions rather than on laws and principles." Then
along came Samuel Hahnemann who "formulated for the first time
in the history of medicine the complete laws and principles govern-

ing health and disease ... and proved them in actual clinical experience."

Though his system worked marvelously, Hahnemann was far ahead of his time. Orthodox medical researchers failed to understand that "both the microbe AND constitutional susceptibility are necessary to initiate disease." This obsession with microbes has lead "to the development of increasingly toxic drugs, which themselves are becoming a significant public health menace."

"The vast majority of drugs," George shows, "are not designed to be curative ... but merely offer the pallid hope of palliation. This in itself is a sign of the helplessness of modern medicine."

What, George asks, should the ideal therapeutic system provide? "It must be effective," he answers, "with ... no risk to the patient and must be based upon ... the enhanced constitutional strength and well-being of the individual.... It should not be prohibitively expensive, and should be readily accessible and understandable to all...."

"What is the objective of human life?" he asks next. "What are we searching for?" His answer is simple. "Everyone seeks an inner state of happiness, a happiness that is unconditional and continuous, a happiness that will depend very little on external conditions."

What It Means to Be Human

In chapter one George begins to lay foundations. "The human organism is not an isolated entity. As with all things, it was originally designed to function harmoniously and compatibly in the environment ... to establish a dynamic balance in which both the individual and the environment are mutually benefited. Any imbalance leads to destruction.... Most people experience degrees of imbalance ... imbalance in the organism's ability to cope with internal and external influences.

"Every organism possesses a defense mechanism which is constantly coping with stimuli from both internal and external sources. Any significant impairment of its function rapidly leads to imbalance and finally death. If the defense mechanism were always functioning perfectly, there would never be any suffering, symptoms or disease. If the stimuli are stronger than the organism's natural resistance (as is usually the case) a state of imbalance is created which then manifests itself as signs and symptoms.

"Although these *effects* are experienced by the entire person, they are expressed with relatively greater force on either mental, emotional or physical levels, depending on the individual's predisposition. Erroneously called diseases, they represent the struggle of the defense mechanism to counteract the morbific (negatively acting) stimulus."

When George speaks of "environmental influences," on the individual, nothing is excluded. His definition encompasses "the universe as a whole...the solar system, the nation, the immediate society, geographical location, the family." And everything affects the state of our health, not just microbes.

So, while orthodox medicine contents itself with the narrow and negative concepts of microbes and disease, homeopathy goes on to consider the equally important idea of "susceptibility," i.e. the degree of strength or weakness of the individual's defense mechanism. This in turn reflects the overall state of his or her health.

Examples of Susceptibility

Consider the effect a very humid climate can have on people with different levels of health. George tells us that....

"1. A quite healthy person's system will resist humidity with minimal disturbance ... and will recover.

2. A person with lesser health may develop stiffness of muscles, pains in the joints, sinusitis ... or asthma. The focus in such a case is primarily on the physical level.

3. A person with worse health may develop anxiety or even depression in such a climate. The focus here is on the emotional level.

4. Someone with very poor health may develop dullness of mind and an inability to concentrate. The focus here is on the mental level."

From this example of the effects of humidity (a purely physical stimulus) George moves dramatically to an example of the dev-

astating emotional effect on a young girl of jealousy and competition from her mother. If the stress continues unabated for a long
time, the daughter is likely to react as follows. . . .

"1. If the daughter is quite healthy, she may eventually disre-
gard and ignore the mother's influence. . . . The stimulus in this
instance has not overcome the organism's natural resistance, and
thus has not created a state of imbalance.

2. If the daughter is not quite so healthy, she may well
develop severe acne on her face, or eczema or duodenal ulcer.
Here the stimulus is stronger than the defense system, but manifests symptoms solely on the physical level.

3. If the daughter's health has been further undermined, a
more serious ailment may develop. In the beginning it may be
excessive lack of confidence in social situations, later apathy, and
finally depression. The manifestation here is emotional.

4. If the daughter's health were further deteriorated, due to
hereditary predisposition, the same stress would overwhelm her
resistance more severely. She might be unable to concentrate in
school or complain that she does not comprehend material which
previously was understood perfectly. Such a progression may well
end in psychosis, because the stress is transmitted to the center of
her being, the mental level.

"Crucial and profound conclusions can be drawn from these
examples. The human being is a whole, integrated entity, not frag-
mented into independent parts (as orthodox medicine would have
us believe. Conventional medicine merely treats symptoms). "If
the liver is affected," it says, "give something for the liver. If the
nose is running, give medicine for the nose."

The Three Dynamic Planes

As we have seen in these examples, symptoms are manifested on
three levels: the physical, the emotional and the mental. At any
given moment, "the activity is *centered* mainly on one of these
planes, but there is always dynamic interaction among the three.
The mental level is most important, and the physical the least, e.g.
a person can be happy and of creative service to himself and others

with a crippled body, blindness or missing limbs, but disturbance on the mental/spiritual level threatens a person's very existence.

"A healthy mind exhibits clarity, coherence and creativity. Confusion, disunity and distraction characterize the completely diseased mind. Selfishness and acquisitiveness are the primary factors that derange the mind. The degree of health or disease of the individual can thus be evaluated from a survey of all three levels."

But there are gradations and priorities established by the body within each level. George calls these "hierarchies." He next provides examples of common mental afflictions ... and the pathological conditions toward which they lead.

Mental Aberrations

"A person who can never express himself clearly, who has great difficulty finding the right words, may eventually enter a state of senility or imbecility. Another individual may have clarity but lacks coherence. He has lost his capacity for abstract thinking and has become subject to impulses. He jumps from subject to subject, perhaps brilliantly, but so rapidly that others are left mystified. Such a person is deeply disturbed on the mental level.

"The master criminal plans a theft or murder with the utmost clarity and rationality, but he is ill in the deepest regions of his being, because he is pursuing selfish goals at the expense of other people. Individuals who are highly egotistical and intolerant pave the way for a state of confusion which may eventually lead to insanity."

So, if the wages of sin is death, the wages of selfishness and greed may be insanity!

"The emotional plane is next in importance. It's imbalances manifest themselves as heightened sensitivity to the sense of ourselves as vulnerable beings separate from the rest of creation (i.e. as selfishness). At the opposite extreme, a oneness with all creation, love, bliss, devotion, etc. characterize the most evolved emotional states. Feelings of inner calm, joy, euphoria, etc. provide the best possible emotional nourishment."

As with the mental state, emotional afflictions are ranked

according to their threat to the individual. Starting with the most threatening, in declining order, George lists suicidal depression, apathy, sadness, anguish, phobias, anxiety, irritability and finally mere dissatisfaction.

The physical plane, though least important, is the only one of the three with which orthodox medicine concerns itself—perhaps explaining why its record of cure is so poor!

As on the other planes, the hierarchy, or order of importance of organs, is vital to evaluating the state of the patient's health, the progression of illness and the effects upon it of any therapy. Despite the vast amount of orthodox medical research, allopathy has ignored this hierarchy, perhaps because it only treats individual symptoms, not the whole patient.

On the physical plane, starting with the most important and working down, George lists the brain, heart, pituitary gland, liver, lungs, kidneys, testes/ovaries, vertebrae and finally the muscles. Homeopaths have learned by experience that, "progressively more serious ailments may be the result of suppression of symptoms of less serious ailments." They know that "if an adverse direction in the hierarchy occurs after treatment, it must be suspected that the therapy is doing harm, not good."

The Homeopath's Measure of Health

George's definition of health serves to summarize what we have learned about ideal conditions on each of the three planes.

"Health in the physical body," he tells us, "is freedom from pain, a state of well-being. On the emotional level it is dynamic serenity: the capability of freely feeling the full range of human emotions without being *enslaved* by them. Health on the mental level is freedom from selfishness. The measurement of health is *creativity*, i.e. all those acts and functions which promote for the individual—and for others —continuous and unconditional happiness."

George next presents diagrams which show how the three levels, each with their hierarchies, are superimposed on one another to form an accurate three dimensional model that will allow the practitioner to sort through the morass of seemingly random and confusing changes in their patients and accurately determine the direction of cure or degeneration.

Case examples show how the body responds to afflictions. For instance, "the two centers of the physical body which correspond most closely to the emotional and mental levels are the heart and the brain."

To illustrate, George tells us of a 19-year old boy who developed excessive stiffness in the back of his neck while preparing for university entrance exams. He had *mentally* decided on a difficult course of study and was *emotionally* reacting to his decision with great anxiety and uncertainty. "The neck seems to be the main pathway connecting the brain and the heart, so it reflected the mental/emotional confict with physical pain in this pathway." The conflict between the two produced a pain in his neck.

We see from this example that "the defense mechanism always attempts to create a wall of defense at the lowest practical level. This level in the individual is called the 'center of gravity' of the disturbance. It may be altered by three factors in the patient:

1. The *hereditary* strength or weakness of the defense mechanism.

2. The *intensity* of the morbific stimuli.

3. The degree of interference caused by *treatments*, e.g. if an allopathic drug is used to relieve pain, the defense mechanism must create a new barrier at a more threatening level to the patient.

Thus, allopathic medicines, which focus upon specific symptoms, actually weaken the defense mechanism and cause a deterioration of health into even more serious chronic diseases."

The Vital Force

The defense mechanism was defined centuries ago by ancients under a philosophy known as "Vitalism." It postulated the presence of a vital force possessing the intelligence and power to govern the myriad processes of both health and disease. Apparently some animating force enters the organism at the time of conception, guides all the functions of life, and then leaves at the time of death. Reflection upon these undeniable facts renders the concept of 'vital force' not only true and understandable but highly appealing. George elaborates....

"Clearly the vital force includes a wide variety of functions, one aspect of which is the balance in states of disease that we call the 'defense mechanism.' The defense mechanism, acting on all three levels of the organism, can be viewed as a tool of the vital force acting in the context of disease.

"New concepts in physics are beginning to be reflected in biological science, particularly in the study of electrodynamic fields of the human body. The vital force possesses all the qualities being discovered by modern research into biological electrodynamic fields ... and more. Master nineteeth century homeopath J.T. Kent, twenty years before Einstein's revolutionary theories, accurately characterized the vital force as having formative intelligence, being subject to change and creating order in the body."

The vital force is synonymous with the electrodynamic field of the body and therefore conforms to known principles of physics. Every substance has a particular resonant frequency at which it will vibrate with greater force when stimulated by a wave of similar frequency.

"The electromagnetic field of the body can be considered its *dynamic plane*, a plane of inconceivable complexity which nevertheless conforms to laws and principles grounded in electromagnetic concepts. These laws and principles are the basis for the new 'energy medicine.'

The Defense Mechanism

"The whole organism, and any component of it, can be strengthened or weakened, depending on the degree of harmony, resonance and the force of the (afflicting or curative) influence applied to it. If the stimulus is stronger than the vital force, the defense mechanism is called into play to counteract it.

"The change on the dynamic plane (i.e. the body's mean vibration rate) is instantaneous, but varying amounts of time may pass before the defense mechanism generates symptoms. This delay is known as the 'incubation period.' During this time, the organism is 'immune' to other similar viruses because the body's resonant frequency has been changed by the inital stimulus."

Once this period has passed, "the susceptibility of the organism to disease is changed, i.e. there is a new spectrum of diseases to which the person is susceptible. That explains familiar cases in which the patient seems to acquire a series of infections of increasing virulence and decreasing responsiveness to antibiotics. Homeopathic physicians are wise enough not to give antibiotics with each new microbe, but instead allow the strengthened defense mechanism to complete the healing process.

Homeopathic Resonance

"The principle of resonance (i.e. of matching vibration levels) renders the organism susceptible on basically only one level at any given moment. In the resulting principle of susceptibility, a person can be 'immune' to gonorrhea either because he is too sick or too healthy (i.e. the vibration rate of his dynamic plane is too high or too low to resonate with the particular frequency of gonorrhea).

"Consider another example. The more psychotic a person is, the less likely that he will acquire an acute (less severe) ailment."

Following the laws of electrodynamic physics, we have seen how negative influences can undermine health by changing the body's vibration rate negatively. But "beneficial influences are also subject to the principle of resonance. Beneficial stimulus, matched to the correct resonant frequency, alters the vibration rate in the direction of greater health. If a curative action occurs, by any therapy, it is because the treatment resonates with the patient's level of susceptibility.

"Herbal treatments, acupuncture, polarity massage, etc, can all produce health benefits when the stimulus happens to match the level of receptivity. With most therapies this occurs by chance, because the resonant frequency of the treatment was not intentionally matched to that of the illness. So such beneficial chance occurrences are rare, and most are later suppressed by drugs or other inappropriate treatment.

"In homeopathy, however, we at last see a scientific system

which is based on clear principles, which aims to stimulate the organism beneficially at precisely the right resonant frequency, and which then allows the strengthened defense mechanism to complete its work properly.

The Dynamic Plane

"The *dynamic plane,* the plane on which disease originates, as well as the plane of the defense mechanism, permeates all levels of the patient. It has exactly the same relationship to the physical body as electromagnetic fields have to matter. Modern cybernetics demonstrate a fundamental principle which applies to the human organism.

"*Any highly organized system always reacts to stress by producing the best possible response of which it is capable at the moment.*"

In other words, our defense mechanisms are always doing their best to protect us from adverse influences of all types. George elaborates. . . .

"In the world today there are only three widely known therapies which can act directly (and thus curatively) on the dynamic plane: acupuncture, the 'laying on of hands' by a spiritually evolved channel for universal energies, and homeopathy. Master acupuncturists and highly evolved spiritual healers are rare. But homeopathy can be learned by any dedicated student in approximately the same amount of time required for allopathic medical training."

So only homeopathy has the potential of producing the large numbers of healers so desperately needed in the world today.

Results Are What Count

"Again and again homeopathy has demonstrated extremely effective curative results in a high percentage of cases, with long-lasting benefits, because it is based on readily comprehensible principles. But how exactly do we go about selecting the therapeutic agent (homeopathic remedy) which can powerfully stimulate the patient's dynamic plane? Symptoms and signs are the only clues. The defense mechanism, in an attempt to heal the organism, produces various signs and symptoms. These are not problems in themselves (as allopaths believe) but simply represent the defense mechanism's best attempt to cure the disturbance.

"To directly affect the patient's dynamic plane, we must find a substance similar enough to its frequency to produce resonance. Since the defense mechanism's only perceptible manifestation is the patient's signs and symptoms, it logically follows that we must seek a homeopathic remedy that can produce in that patient a similar totality of signs and symptoms.

"If the substance can produce a similar symptom picture in a healthy person, then the likelihood is good that its vibration rate will be close to the frequency of the diseased person. Therefore a powerful strengthening of the defense mechanism can occur—through the homeopathic principle of resonance.

"The fundamental pillar of homeopathy is *like cures like*. Or as Samuel Hahnemann, the founder of homeopathy, stated it: *Any substance which can produce a totality of symptoms in a healthy human being, can cure that totality of symptoms in a sick human being.*"

This startling principle, called The Law of Similars, is the backbone of homeopathy. It runs exactly counter to the disastrous view of orthodox medicine, which insists that symptoms are evil and must immediately be eradicated at any cost.

As George puts it, "Conventional doctors do not respect the symptom as an attempt of the body to heal. Therefore their therapeutics are not designed to strengthen the defense mechanism.

"Allopaths take a cursory look at gross and obvious symptoms and hunt for a microbe, without bothering to consider the patient's susceptibility. The homeopath carefully studies the *totality* of the symptoms and is relatively uninterested in the nature of the microbe. He searches for a substance that reflects as closely as possible the total picture of the patient's symptoms.

"The symptoms of most importance to the homeopath are those which most highly individualize the particular patient. Only by such refinement is it possible to approach with precision the true resonant frequency of both the patient and the remedy, which in turn can lead to cure."

Finding the Match

Matching the patient's total symptom picture to the known symptom picture of a particular remedy will produce the resonance required to effect a cure. That's why the homeopath takes such pains and probes so deeply into the patient's symptoms. He must "record the totality of all deviations from normal on all three levels (physical, mental and emotional) to discover the complete and individual symptom picture of his patient."

So, in addition to asking questions about the patient's prime complaints, he will probe the patient's tolerance to heat and cold, the effects of humidity and weather changes, times of day when the patient feels worse, the effects of all foods, including strong cravings and aversions, favored positions for sleeping and the degree of sleeping comfort, anxieties, phobias and irritabilities and the circumstances that produce them, how the mind functions in various situations . . . and so on.

The answers to all these questions will gradually produce an individual symptom picture in the mind of the homeopath . . . a picture that he must match to the proven picture of a particular homeopathic remedy.

There are many hundreds of remedies which have been fully proved, and thousands more that are partially proved. Homeopathic remedies may be animal, mineral or vegetable, so long as they are biologically active substances, open to electromagnetic interaction with the body. They may have beneficial or highly toxic effects on the body. The individual's specific reaction depends on his degree of susceptibility or 'affinity' for the substance. Even the crude (unprepared) form of a substance may be therapeutic temporarily, but it is also likely to produce toxic side effects in the patient.

Potentization

Two hundred years ago Hahnemann found that diluting the substance reduced the toxicity—but also reduced the therapeutic effects. Then he somehow discovered that adding kinetic energy to his dilutions by violent shaking or 'succussion,' *increased* their potency while reducing the toxicity. It was a major medical discovery, solving two problems simultaneously. He wrote,

"The more a substance is succussed and diluted, the greater the therapeutic effect while simultaneously nullifying the toxic effects."

There appears to be no limit to this natural law. The greater the dilution, the greater the potency—so long as succussion accompanies dilution.

Allopaths have always resisted this assertion, despite undeniable clinical evidence, because it runs contrary to old-fashioned beliefs, and because traditional chemistry (Avogadro's Law) insists that beyond a dilution of 24x (or 12c), there is no chance of a molecule of the original substance remaining in solution. That is somewhat like comparing apples and oranges. Avogadro's law does not seem to apply because homeopathic dilutions are energized with succussion. In adding kinetic energy, succussion perfectly fits the electromagnetic theory of homeopathy. George explains....

"Why this occurs is not thoroughly understood. Apparently the energy contained in the original substance is somehow released by succussion and transmitted to the molecules of the solvent, i.e. distilled water. The water molecules then take on the dynamic energy of the original substance. A hundred years of clinical results all over the world confirm that the water molecules still retain the 'vibrational frequency' of the original substance, but the energy has been enhanced to such a vast degree that it is capable of stimulating the dynamic plane of the patient sufficiently to produce a cure."

Consider a typical example. "A patient whose symptom picture resonates with that of Belladonna will respond to just a few drops of Belladonna tincture, but the response to this low a potency may be minimal and short-acting. A 12c potency (diluted 100/1 twelve times) will probably produce more dramatic relief. If a 10,000c potency is administered, the response will likely be a complete disappearance of all symptoms within a matter of hours, with no relapse whatever." In other words, a cure.

"So, to obtain curative results that are lasting, it is necessary to increase the intensity of the electromagnetic field of the remedy through potentization, i.e. simultaneous succussion and dilution.

"Neither one nor the other alone is effective. Remedies potentized by dilution and succussion are unique to homeopathy—and uniquely curative when the symptom picture of the remedy matches that of the patient, producing electromagnetic resonance.

The Major Threats

"Thus far the human organism has been depicted as an integrated totality, responding to external stimuli by a change in vibration rate on the electromagnetic level. If the defense mechanism is weak or the stimulus is powerful, the vibration rate will alter for the worse. We therefore potentize remedies to strengthen their electromagnetic level and prescribe them according to Hahnemann's Law of Similars, to take advantage of the resonance between the remedy and the vibration level of the human organism.

"The most powerful *negative* influences which can deeply and chronically alter health are:

1. Acute illness.
2. Suppressive therapies (especially allopathic drugs).
3. Vaccinations.

The health level of the human organism will not jump upward or downward without the impact of powerful influences. A healthy person will not suddenly become psychotic, and a psychotic individual is unlikely to spontaneously become mentally and emotionally healthy. However, an acute illness to which the individual is very susceptible can also seriously alter his level of health.

"Allopathic drugs produce adverse shocks to the human organism, because they are prescribed solely for local symptoms, ignoring the totality of the patient's symptom picture."

Allopathic drugs produce a symptomatic response from the defense mechanism that allopaths refer to as "side-effects." Actually, these side-effects "represent the defense mechanism's best effort to counteract the undesireable stimulus of the drug. To the body these drugs are diseases in themselves."

Hahenemann, almost two hundred years ago, put it even more strongly. . . .

"*These devastations and maimings of the human organism . . . with harmful drugs and treatment must be remedied by the vital force ... if it has not already been too much weakened by such mischievous acts. These inroads on human health are the most deplorable, the most incurable of all chronic diseases."*

If this was true in Hahnemann's time, think how much more true it must be today, with modern medicine's vast arsenal of untested overpowering drugs! George expands.

The Worst Drugs

"Drugs of all types, of course, are damaging, but the most disturbing to the human organism are antibiotics, tranquilizers, contraceptive pills, cortisone and other hormones. But literally *any* drug can be disruptive if the person is susceptible to it. Thus we see people having fatal reactions to minute doses of penicillin, aspirin and other supposedly mild drugs. *Since allopathic drugs are never selected according to the Law of Similars, they inevitably superimpose a new drug disease which then must be counteracted by the organism.*

"The human organism is weakened and disturbed by drugs in two ways: (1) by the influence of the drug itself, and (2) by interference with the defense mechanism. The real tragedy is that the defense mechanism, once poisoned, cannot then reestablish the original equilibrium of the body on its own. Paradoxically, people weakened by allopathic drugs become relatively 'protected' from certain infections and epidemics, but this is a sign of their degenerated health, not of improvement.

"The allopathic community likes to boast that acute diseases have diminished in this century." Ironically, that's partially because allopathic drugs have weakened the population to the point of immunity!

"While acute diseases have declined," George tells us, "there has been a corresponding increase in such vastly more crippling chronic diseases as cancer, heart disease, strokes, neurological disorders, epilepsy, violence, insanity," and now immune difficiency afflictions like AIDS.

The Dangers of Vaccination

Even more insidious than allopathic drugs are current government programs of vaccination, because they are forced on the entire population, and because trusting people are led to believe that vaccination is both safe and essential to the general welfare. The so-called "benefits" alledgedly conferred by vaccination are often cited as one of the major "successes" of modern medicine. Nothing could be farther from the truth! Homeopaths recognize vaccination as a potent threat to the health and even the lives of a majority of the population! Listen to George on the subject....

"Vaccines are administered to entire populations without any consideration of individuality and regardless of the state of health or individual susceptibility. Not surprisingly, in a high percentage of cases, vaccination has a profoundly disturbing effect on health, particularly in relation to chronic disease. A vaccine tends to negatively change the electromagnetic vibration rate in the same way as a severe illness or allopathic drug." There are basically five different responses to vaccinaton . . . none of them beneficial!

1. No response because the system is too healthy.

2. No response because of deep constitutional weakness. Neither of these cases are benefited by vaccination, since they cannot contract the threatening disease anyway, because their vibration levels are too far removed from it.

3. A mild reaction indicates the individual is susceptible, but his defense mechanism is not strong enough to overcome the effect of the vaccine. It's noxious influence then remains in the body, and the vibration rate of the person is negatively altered.

4. If the vaccine produces a strong reaction, with fever and other systemic symptoms, then the defense mechanism is probably strong enough to overcome the negative influence of the vaccine. But the individual is still susceptible to the threatening disease and may well contract it if exposed, despite vaccination!

5. A very strong reaction, such as encephalitis, meningitis or paralysis, means the individual's suceptibility is quite high but the defense mechanism is too weak to counteract the vaccine, so a

deep illness is produced. In this tragic circumstance, the patient's health may be permanently impaired.

"Any chronic condition which can be traced to vaccination is called *vaccinosis*. It is often found by homeopaths to follow administration of rabies, measles, polio, influenza, typhoid, paratyphoid, DPT and even tetanus vaccines. Many cases of vaccinosis are dramatically benefited by administration of a potentized homeopathic preparation of the particular vaccine used.

"For instance, a 50-year old woman was homeopathically cured of hay fever—until she received a smallpox vaccination prior to foreign travel. Her reaction to the vaccine was mild but her hay fever returned immediately. She was then more difficult to treat homeopathically, but eventually order was reestablished in her system.

"Homeopaths are convinced that vaccination is a large-scale factor in the degenerating health of our populations. There are numerous examples. For instance, our government made a major effort recently to vaccinate the entire population against an expected epidemic of swine flu. The epidemic never materialized, but of the 50 million Americans vaccinated, 581 developed a (crippling) paralytic neurological disorder. This represented a sevenfold increase in that disease over the population at large! Such disastrous consequences are predictable when a foreign substance is injected into large numbers of people without regard for individual susceptibility."

As the truth about vaccination spreads, trust in government-sponsored vaccination programs is rapidly deteriorating. More and more thoughtful parents are legally refusing to have their small children innoculated. They simply invoke their right to reject vaccination on the basis of philosophical or religious belief. This vital subject is treated more fully in chapter 14.

"In addition to vaccination, acute illness and drugs, there is one other major factor in susceptibility to disease: heredity."

Hereditary Susceptibility

Susceptibility to chronic disease is often inherited. We have already seen that "disease cannot occur without both an *exciting cause* and a *maintaining cause.* The exciting cause may be a microorganism, an allopathic drug, an emotional shock, a vaccination, a chemical or similar stimulus. The maintaining cause is susceptibility or 'predisposition' to chronic disease, which is very largely hereditary.

"DNA is only part of the story. Ailments can be transmitted to children by means of the parents' electrodynamic field at the time of conception, even though no genetic change has occured in the parents. In this way, their predisposition to chronic disease can be inherited. The predisposition produced in the child is a combination of the individual predispositions of the parents, reflecting both their general health and their specific state of health *at the moment of conception.* Prospective parents should therefore do everything possible to maximize their health during child-bearing years, to save their children tremendous amounts of suffering throughout life.

"Hahnemann discovered that the vast majority of patients have been weakened through hereditary influence, drugs or vaccinations, resulting in several layers of predisposition." These must be treated one at a time, starting with the outermost, before a cure is complete. "The prescriber systematically peels off layer after layer of predisposing weaknesses by carefully prescribing each remedy based on the totality of symptoms in view at the moment."

This ticklish job requires a highly trained and experienced homeopath skilled in constitutional prescribing ... like the physicians at Hahnemann Clinic. It should not be attempted by lay prescribers, no matter how deft. George explains why.

"A remedy given at the wrong time either has no effect or creates damage of two types: it can interfere with progress toward a cure, and it can disorder the defense mechanism enough to complicate and confuse the case."

George provides several clinical examples which involve my own beloved remedy, Tuberculinum. He says, "Cancer, tuberculosis and other major illnesses transmit characteristic disease-images from one generation to another. For example, the child of a parent with tuberculosis may not get tuberculosis, *per se,* but is likely to suffer from asthmatic bronchitis, hay fever, sinusitis, etc. All these are manifest in the provings of Tuberculinum, which is a potentized 'nosode' prepared from an actual tubercular abscess.

"In the same manner, a patient may acquire a chronic disease disposition after a bout with a severe infectious disease, and this predisposition may then be transmitted to subsequent generations. Allopathic drugs and vaccinations can have the same effect. Smallpox vaccination, rabies vaccine, polio immunization, cortisone, penicillin and tranquilizers are all capable of weakening the defense mechanism sufficiently to predispose the individual who takes them to chronic diseases of many types."

A Tuberculinum Case Example

Finally comes a clinical example of inherited predispositions from one of George's multi-layer patients.

"A young man had suffered recurrent episodes of asthmatic bronchitis for many years. A variety of homeopathic remedies had effectively relieved his acute attacks, but relief had not been long lasting. After two years it became clear that the youth's fundamental predisposition had not been curatively affected by the remedies. It was, however, noted that he showed some symptoms of Tuberculinum and one of his parents had had tuberculosis.

"When Tuberculinum was given, the attacks of asthmatic bronchitis dramatically decreased, finally disappearing altogether.

"But after two years he began to experience bursitis in his right shoulder and arthritis in his left shoulder and right knee. These new symptoms were relieved by various homeopathic remedies, but again the cures were not lasting. Gradually an underlying layer, less deep than the first, became apparent to the homeopath. Its picture showed indications of Calcarea carbonica. The remedy was given and the patient was cured.

"Each remedy in this case had been prescribed on the totality of symptoms evident at the moment, but during acute attacks the acute symptoms had lead to relatively superficial remedies. Rarely can a remedy be found which covers *every* detailed symptom of the patient. There are always a few minor symptoms which don't fit and must therefore be temporarily disregarded. But over a period of time, when the case is reviewed, these may lead us to the deeper acting remedy."

That concludes my condensation of the 135 pages of Section 1, "The Laws and Principles of Cure" in George's admirable textbook. Section 2, "The Principles of Homeopathy in Practical Application" is even more fascinating but increasingly complex. Excerpts, however, from George's Introduction may further intrigue the reader.

"The concepts in Section 1 are merely sterile ideas until tested in the arena of clinical experience. In their application the profound truths of homeopathy become alive with meaning and vivid in action. Once the underlying principles have been understood we must plunge into the *art* of homeopathy. The actual process of prescribing demands a full understanding of the fundamental laws and principles which must be fused in an artistic manner into a unique application for each patient.

"The prescriber becomes an intimate participant in the life of the patient, sympathetic and sensitive as well as objective and accepting. Experience in the deepest regions of human existence is gained, which stimulates growth in the prescriber, just as it does in the patient."

The book concludes with Appendix B, an intriguing condensation, complete with diagrams, of 22 sample clinical cases showing evaluations one month after initial prescribing. These condensed accounts read like character sketches for suspenseful psychological fiction, and they admirably illustrate the difficult art of extracting symptom pictures from unique individuals and matching them to the remedies that will cure.

The Science of Homeopathy by George Vithoulkas is available in paper at this writing from Grove Press for $12.50.

3

Understanding Homeopathic Mysteries

An Illuminating Phone Follow-Up ... Homeopathic
Musings... Disaster in the Desert ... Exile in the Snow ...
Mom Gets Poisoned ... Back to the Clinic ... Suppressing
My Fungus ... Eye Trouble Discovered ... Post Mortem ...
Looking Toward Hawaii

When a month had passed since my followup visit, I paddled across
the lake to the pay phone to report to Dr. Gray. He was encouraged. "Yours is a typical reaction," he told me. "In the next few
months you may see a return of symptoms you experienced as a
teenager or child."

"And I never get to treat them?"

He chuckled. "We don't like to say 'never.' If you feel you have
to have some relief, go ahead, but you're better off without it.
Think of it this way. Your vital force has been stimulated by the
remedy you took. It's working hard to cure you. These symptoms
reveal its efforts to rid your body of toxins."

That seemed clear.

"Anything you do to suppress symptoms thwarts the vital force
and delays the treatment, because it has to undo whatever suppression takes place. So if you put something on your brow, it would
probably cause an inflammation like the Vaseline did. But worst of
all it would mean a setback, a delay. Before you could progress, the

vital force would have to throw off the suppression so it could get back to the job of ridding the body of toxins."

"So, letting my symptoms run their course is what cures me?"

"That's exactly how it works. But I think you'll soon notice improvements, too. For instance, when this is done, you won't need Vaseline any more."

It didn't seem possible. Vaseline had always been essential to my life.

Bill explained. "You see, the symptoms you experience are the body's way of permanently removing the effects of suppression back over the years. Your body's trying to get back in balance. Unfortunately, if you give it a crutch, it'll use it. Once you get past all the suppression, you'll get better. But first the suppressive influence must be removed."

I paddled back across the lake to the cabin for lunch, thinking about our conversation. Bill had forecast the eruption of more symptoms, but he also predicted noticeable improvement. Was that a contradiction? Could I get better and worse at the same time? Apparently I could. After all, the redness and itching that had afflicted my face for years was greatly improved. So was the heart-burn at night.

Homeopathy had done a lot for me already. And I had to admire its bold simplicity and systematic theory. There were no loose ends or vague presumptions. I liked the orderliness and stability. There was also great appeal in the holistic nature of the treatment. I had always been suspicious, I realized, of attempts to get rid of a single symptom without regard for the rest of the body—not to mention the patient's mental and emotional aspects. How vastly more sensible it seemed to think of curing the whole organism, instead of settling for "temporary symptomatic relief."

Mild, safe homeopathic remedies could apparently unleash the almost frightening power of the genie that lives within all of us, a mysterious inner energy known as the vital force. I often found myself wondering about this sleeping giant that could be energized by just the right magic potion. As far as I could tell, I was taking this grand adventure completely without risk. I might suffer 'aggravations' and feel anxiety about what was to come, but my body was in absolutely no danger. The remedies were all completely non-toxic.

But the greatest appeal I had found in homeopathy was its potential for bringing greater happiness by curing mental and emotional afflictions! If negative symptoms like anger, anxiety, frustration and insecurity could be cured, the door would be open to greater personal happiness!

But it was also clear that homeopathy isn't for everyone. It's too different, too strange and—for many—too slow. And on a minority of patients it simply doesn't work. No one knows why. It requires self-discipline, understanding, restraint, self-denial and patience. And it doesn't much help that establishment medicine—county medical societies, doctors, the AMA and the billion dollar drug industry—all do their best to discredit it, to keep it strange, suspect and relatively unknown.

Some aspects of homeopathy are just plain hard to believe. Like the fact that homeopathic remedies become more potent as they become more dilute. Though thoroughly proven by results for two centuries, the notion runs contrary to everything we've been taught since we were children. And many Americans won't have enough respect for their bodies to choose homeopathy. The average patient, I'm afraid, given a choice between the trauma of major surgery and powerful dangerous drugs on the one hand, and a three year harmless cure with only aggravations to deal with on the other, would probably elect for surgery and drugs—because the procedure is fast and familiar! In America, the quick fix is king—even if it doesn't last!

Two days after talking to Bill my crusty brow mysteriously cleared up. After two months of chafing, peeling and crusting, it was as smooth and clear as a baby's bottom! Believing I had worked my way through the remedy's facial symptoms, I got cocky. I began to wash my face again, and now when my brow itched I no longer restrained myself from scratching.

The honeymoon was over in four days! Within a week my face was back where it started, and my crotch rash, after nearly disappearing, returned. But I didn't really mind. Symptoms were evidence that the remedy was still working. I was consoled by the thought that these strange extrusions were manifestations of my revitalized "vital force," rebelling against the vain efforts of physicians for fifty-five years to suppress my symptoms. I now thought of the various excrescences on my skin as a distillate of all the poisons and foreign substances I'd ever taken into my body—like the slime cooked out of the skin in a sauna.

On September first, my fifty-fifth birthday, we drove home to the desert, arriving in late afternoon. School began the next day for our six-year-old daughter, Angela. The sea of sage surrounding the house hadn't yet blossomed but the yellow blooms of rabbit brush were everywhere! Nevertheless, I decided to spend a few nights. The next day dawned cold and rainy with a black threatening sky. I knew it would be stormier at Echo, maybe snowing, so I decided to stay another day. That afternoon I began to experience intense itching in my crotch, and my nose grew congested. By dark I was convulsively sneezing and my nose was running like a fountain.

The next morning I was desperate to escape. I didn't care if it was snowing at Echo! All that mattered was getting away from the tormenting pollen! I think I would have killed to escape it! Irritably, with running nose and streaming swollen eyes, I kissed my wife goodbye and left. My eyes were weeping so heavily I could hardly see through the windshield. Half an hour later in the mountains I felt better, but back at the cabin, my symptoms came back. The attack lasted an hour, then suddenly stopped. For the next four days I experienced periodic episodes of weeping and sneezing, but gradually they grew shorter and less frequent. The fall weather at Echo continued cold and stormy. I was cut off from my home and family by my allergy. I felt exiled, marooned, like Napoleon on Elba. But there was plenty of time to sit by the fire and ponder homeopathy's problems ... like the difficulty of gaining credibility for its cures.

Every establishment, by definition, gets to set the standards by which its competitors are judged. Medicine is no exception. Take flu drugs for example. Since allopathy simplistically classifies people into broad disease categories, it decrees that the efficacy of any flu drug must be tested by taking 200 people with the flu and doing double blind tests, giving some placebo and some the flu drug.

But homeopathy works by treating the whole organism, not just flu symptoms. And it does so on an individual not a group basis. So homeopathy can never satisfy the allopathic criteria—and that's exactly how the allopathic establishment wants it! Homeopathy's best answer is its undeniable success—especially when accurately compared to allopathy's dismal failures. Ultimately, I believe, the public will respond to a system that is proven to work consistently, inexpensively and safely—even if the medical establishment jealously or ignorantly disapproves.

When a foot and half of snow fell in less than two days, turning summer into winter, I gathered my dirty laundry and drove back to the desert to see my family and get warm. But I vowed I wouldn't stay more than one night. I wouldn't risk turning into a pumpkin! As usual, I felt great for the first few hours, although the sage was now in blossom along with the rabbit brush. That night it snowed and Deanne argued that the pollen would be soaked and plastered to the sand, so why didn't I try a second night? I was tempted, but I left while I still felt good.

On the return trip to Echo my symptoms all came back. Was it delayed reaction or the pollen I'd brought with me, or something else? I soon had the answer. Every night I sat reading by the fire in a beanbag covered with a raw wool Indian blanket. And every night I sneezed. Then one night I got up and put the blanket outside, replacing it with a cotton flannel sheet. Within minutes my sneezing stopped. Clearly, my body's battle with the desert pollens had sensitized it to other irritants, like cat dander, cigarette smoke . . . and raw wool.

One night I made the trip across the lake to the phone shack in the woods to call my mother, Helen, an active artist-writer of 80 in Berkeley. I was shocked to hear she had just gotten out of the hospital. A week before, when she complained of excess heart pains to her Kaiser Hospital allopathic doctor, he gave her a strong tranquilizer called Elavil. She had told him she didn't want to be doped, but he assured her she needn't worry. "You'll love it," he told her. "Everybody does."

"It turned me into a zombie!" she told me. "I couldn't work. I couldn't even get around the house by myself. I actually had to be led!"

After cutting the dose in half for three straight days, she threw the rest away. When she went back to Kaiser another doctor gave her cortisone. He said it would bring instant relief, but he warned her that it was powerful and might produce side effects. Thinking only of the promised relief, she took it. That evening she suffered multiple heart pains and had to be taken to the hospital in an ambulance. She spent the night in the emergency ward.

"I told them it had to be the cortisone," she told me. "But everyone insisted it just couldn't be. It was like some kind of conspiracy among the nurses to protect the doctors."

She was bewildered because, like most of her generation, she'd always trusted doctors implicitly. This widespread trust of doctors, I believe, is what makes them a greater menace to society as "drug dealers" than the pushers lounging on street corners!

I urged mom to go see Bill Gray at Hahnemann Clinic. "His remedies are safe and effective. They certainly wouldn't put you in the hospital!"

"Oh. I couldn't afford it. It doesn't cost me anything to go to Kaiser. It's all covered by insurance. Anyplace else I'd have to pay."

"Go see him and *I'll* pay," I offered.

"I'll think about it," she said vaguely. "But I'm probably too old to try something new."

It was now mid-September and there was still a month to go before my next date with Bill. We planned to move to Hawaii for the winter but our house there was rented until early November. In a month the basin would be closed for the winter, but I couldn't go home to the desert and its pollen. Where could I spend the three weeks in between? Then Deanne arrived for the weekend with the solution. Our rental agent in Hawaii had phoned to report that our tenant had skipped. Suddenly we were free to reclaim our house. The three problem weeks had disappeared.

I called the Clinic to move up my appointment with Bill. Two weeks later I was back in his office, relating what had happened in the pollen. When I told him about a strange rash in my crotch that kept getting worse, he asked to see it. I stood up and dropped my pants. He leaned across the desk to take a look. "Oh, oh!" he grimaced. "That's a fungus." He studied my array of blisters, frowning. "That may not be the work of the remedy at all."

After questioning me closely about my energy and spirits, he assured me the Tuberculinum was still working well. "So I won't prescribe anything. Just keep doing what you're doing. Avoiding suppression is still the name of the game. You *will* keep getting better and better."

"What about this redness in my crotch?"

He frowned thoughtfully. "I think you should suppress that. Hawaii is very humid. A fungus like this could be very bad over there ... even though you have a healthy vital force. So get some Tinactin and put it on four times a day. Try to get rid of the rash before you go."

I was delighted. I had no idea what was waiting in Hawaii! "If the Tinactin works," I asked, "does that show it wasn't the Tuberculinum, after all?"

"Yes, providing you don't feel worse overall. In homeopathic theory, getting an infection requires a combination of a virulent bacteria *and* a susceptible individual. Allopaths just try to kill the bacteria. We try to strengthen the patient's resistance. The skin is the most superficial manifestation of the defense mechanism, so there isn't much risk in suppressing a skin symptom. It's a reasonable gamble because you're going to Hawaii and you have a strong vital force. If you had a weak vital force I'd say you musn't suppress. Maybe I'd even say you shouldn't go to Hawaii."

"Not go to Hawaii?"

"Some homeopaths would advise you not to, but I believe the patient should live a normal life. For you that means going to Hawaii for the winter. What we're doing here comes under the heading of 'management,' which means bending the rules to fit the circumstances. Here, look at my notes." He handed them across the desk."

"I can't read them without my glasses."

"Oh? You have vision troubles, too?"

"No. Like most people, when I turned forty-five, I needed reading glasses. That's all."

"That's not normal. The remedy should eventually improve your eyesight."

"*Really?* I thought glasses were almost inevitable."

"No, deteriorating eyesight isn't normal. I've been treating a little girl who's almost completely blind. In a year and a half I've gotten her four times the vision her pediatric opthamologist considered possible. Now the woman wants to send me *all* her patients! So, use your reading glasses as little as possible. They're suppressive, too, I'm afraid." He took back his interview notes.

"Do you see a second layer to my case or will the Tuberculium cure me?"

"That depends on the strength of your vital force. Some people's vital force is so strong that they stay the same all through life. There's no second layer. There's only the one remedy. But that's rare. Less than ten percent of Americans. Your vital force is nine on a scale of ten. A real sick person of fifty-five might have five or six layers. You probably have one or two. Your good health made diagnosis hard."

"How did you check me out mentally and emotionally?"

"At first it was just impressions ... what you were like, how you held your body, how you talked, how quickly you opened up, how you interacted, and how interested you were in things. I used all that to measure the strength of your vital force on the mental and emotional planes, as well as on the physical."

"Pretty slick! Over the phone you said my cure would take three years—before you even met me. But the books talk mostly about quick cures."

"Quick cures are for acute conditions, not chronic. Three years is a long average for chronic cures. Actually it's more like two years, but I have to play it safe. If it takes longer than I predict, you might get discouraged."

I nodded. "I thought I might be better this season. I guess I was too optimistic. . . ."

"Exactly!" he laughed. "Tuberculinum *is* optimistic ... or melancholic. When their optimism is dashed, they're miserable. I mean suicidal! There's no point in living. You haven't seen the dark side of Tuberculinum. That's how you would have ended up at age seventy-five or eighty. But now you're protected against that fate."

"I hope so! What do you see happening in Hawaii?"

"It all depends on what the climate change does to your skin. We'll try to cure your crotch rash beforehand. Your brow might get worse, but then it should recover on its own. Your eyes may get worse, but overall you'll be much better, so you shouldn't be distracted. Removing suppressions is like peeling the skin off an onion. With each layer that's removed, you get healthier. Wait and see. You'll get incrementally better over the next six months."

"What medicines are safe to use?"

"The rule of thumb is, as long as you don't expect a medicine to do anything, it's okay to use it." He chuckled at my obvious confusion. "It's really very simple. Any condition that's going to disappear on its own, you can safely treat. It's okay, for instance, to take aspirin for a cold because it's not a lasting affliction. You can treat that kind of thing as you normally would."

"You mean, anything not caused by the Tuberculinum?"

"Correct. Everyday we're exposed to all sorts of stresses— viruses, injuries, fungus—and it's okay to treat them. You're going to be exposed to much more fungus over there."

Those, it turned out, were prophetic words!

Outside in the hall we parted for six months. The first thing I did was buy a tube of Tinactin at the drug store and liberally apply it to my angry red crotch, launching what I hoped would be a swift recovery. There were just three weeks before we left for Hawaii. For the first few days my crotch steadily improved. Then I hit some sort of plateau. I stopped getting better, though I tried every medicine Deanne could find in the drugstore. But the itching was negligible in the cool mountain dryness and it was easy to be philosophic. My Tuberculinum optimism told me it wouldn't matter if a little rash remained.

4

Eminent Homeopaths

Bill Gray MD ... Maesimund Panos MD ...
Roger Morrison MD ... Master George Vithoulkas ... The
Founding of Hahnemann Clinic ... The Homeopath's
Definition of Health

Bill Gray

The eldest son of a nurse and a test pilot, Bill Gray was born in Norfolk, Virginia, on October 13, 1942. His earliest memory—he must have been about four—still fascinates him.

"One day I figured out that other people weren't just extensions of myself," he explains. "Every individual, I suddenly realized, had his or her own complete and magnificent universe, just like me! The discovery simply blew me away! From that day on there was nothing else in the world half so interesting to me as other people. I had an insatiable need to know what they were like, how they felt. I wanted to get into their universes. It was almost an obsession."

When Bill was five, the Grays moved to Los Angeles where his father was working for NASA to develop new planes. Even as a six year old, his mother remembers, Bill would listen so intently and sympathetically to adult neighbors who came to visit that they tended to treat him like another adult. "They seemed to feel he understood them," she says.

By the time he was eight Bill realized that going into medicine would best serve his fascination with getting to know and understand other people. Because his sense of mission came so young, he had highly idealistic feelings about what being a doctor meant. It meant healing and curing ... nothing less!

During his high school years he did a lot of volunteer work in his spare time. He soon found he liked hospitals best. At Los Angeles County Hospital he was the first male Candy-striper, and he organized a support group for Dr. Tom Dooley, one of his early heroes.

"Working with the patients in L.A. County Hospital, I discovered the real appeal of dealing with the sick. People who are suffering, I soon learned, are honest. People in daily life hide behind a facade, but when they're really sick it's different. Who they really are—good, bad or indifferent—comes out. And that's what I was interested in: what those people were really like. Medicine permitted me to be a voyeur, to see into other people's universes."

Once he'd found the path, Bill followed it relentlessly, making his way through high school and U.C.L.A.—where he obtained a degree in microbiology—on the way to prestigious Stanford Medical School.

Then came the big letdown. In medical school he quickly discovered that once he put on the doctor's white coat the facades came up, instead of letting down. Neither he nor his patients were human any more.

"But worst of all," he remembers, "was being put in a position where I had to lie about who *I* was. When you put on that white coat, you have to play doctor, even if you don't know a thing.

"I'll never forget the first time that happened. I was only a student, but the professor introduced me to this woman with severe lupus erythematosis as "her doctor!" She had gone through all kinds of hell in a private hospital out in the sticks, and she'd been sent down to our big city medical center for expert diagnosis and treament! She had a terrible chronic disease, and she was desperate for answers. I didn't know a thing about her disease, but I was 'her doctor.' I was supposed to comfort and diagnose a distraught and dying woman—just for practice!

"She said to me, 'Dr. Gray, I'm really confused and befuddled.

What *is* this disease? How do you diagnose it? How will you treat it?' I didn't know any of the answers, but I couldn't tell her that. She'd have panicked if she ever found out I was only a medical student. So I was forced to lie, and I did. I made up stuff to keep her from freaking out. And I felt *sick* about it!"

Medical schools have changed very little from the beginning of the century. What goes on there is often disgusting, brutal, sadistic and barbaric. No wonder allopathy is failing and dishonesty, on one level or another, is rampant among today's allopathic physicians.

"Students are made to sacrifice their honesty," says Bill, "in order to get through medical school. They are deliberately run into the ground, forced to work past the point of exhaustion and deprived of needed food and sleep. I call that torture! I wouldn't wish it on my worst enemy.

"But the deliberate deceit that's taught is worse. They might as well teach a course in lying! Instead, they force you to lie by making you misrepresent yourself. They feed you false logic. They teach you that it's unkind to tell the patient the truth, so you must lie. They teach you that you can't ever admit you 'don't know,' so you lie. And students are systematically blinded by their professors against the possibility that there's any other way to cure.

"Once you've bought that, it becomes very easy to rationalize. You say, 'If this is the only medicine in the world that will help, we've got to prescribe it, even if it produces disastrous side effects.' They never find out in medical school that other kinds of healing are vastly more effective.

"And later, most of them don't want to find out. They've made an enormous investment of time, money, energy and personal suffering. They don't want to hear that it was wasted or wrong. They don't want to know there's a better way. So they become geniuses at rationalizing. They don't want to hear about allopathy's failures—even if they can't pay their malpractice insurance premiums anymore!

"I call medical school a spiritual battleground for your very soul. It's incredibly difficult to survive it without compromising your honesty! I was lucky. I got mine back! As a kid, I learned a very direct kind of honesty from my parents. Without that, I might have accepted the dishonesty taught me in med school. I might not even have noticed it!"

And the treatment available to the ill, Bill discovered, was appallingly ineffective and dangerous. He found himself surrounded by suffering he couldn't begin to alleviate.

"Anyone who was honest," he says, "could see that conventional medicine was mostly bullshit. It wasn't curing anyone. Most of the time we were helpless. And the side effects were terrible! The toxicity of the drugs we were using were *putting* people in the hospitals, not getting them out!"

Bill was sadly disillusioned to find that forty-five percent of a doctor's time in a hospital is spent dealing with drug complications, not with healing. The only thing he liked about medicine was childbirth. He was absolutely crazy about delivering babies, especially natural childbirth at home, with all the family around. The circumstances were joyful because pregnant women aren't sick!

"It's the favorite thing in my whole life," he beams. "When a woman is having a baby, all her facade, all her defenses, have to fall away. There comes a moment when she's totally real and honest, completely herself. I think it's wonderful to be there, inside that special universe. I still put delivering babies ahead of everything else."

Delivering babies—and pride—were the only things that kept him going in medical school. He almost dropped out of Stanford in his junior year because he knew conventional medicine was all wrong. But his father, who'd done a lot of dangerous flying in his day, talked him into staying.

"His example guided me," Bill recalls. "He explained that sometimes you need to see something through, just to prove you can do it. If you quit, your self-esteem may be shot for life. If I hadn't stayed, I would never have known if I could make it. So I stuck it out."

Bill didn't bother to attend his graduation, and he made himself go through internship at Oakland's Highland hospital just to finish the job, qualify to practice as an M.D. and complete his education.

"Once that was over I said, 'Okay, that's it. I'm not going to do this anymore!' I was ready to chuck medicine altogether and look for another way of satisfying my old dream. Then I remembered chiropractic."

During his internship an orthopedic surgeon had showed him that chiropractic adjustments could provide dramatic and immediate cures. He saw the surgeon cure whiplash patients fresh from automobile wrecks by deftly cracking their necks in the operating room. This simple act saved them from the slow, dreary and often unsuccessful conventional treatment of braces, traction, casts, drugs and hospitalization ... often for many months!

"Now all at once I realized that chiropractic was a totally non-toxic way of treating people," says Bill. "You really can't do lasting damage if you know anything about what you're doing. I also realized I had a built-in prejudice against it! The prejudice had come from my medical training!"

Bill finished his internship in 1971—and immediately dropped out of the system. To support himself he worked at Kaiser Hospital in Oakland as a drop-in clinic doctor, but all his free time was devoted to the search for what he really wanted to do with his life. After the discovery of his prejudice against chiropractic, he realized he probably had others. After all, medical schools teach, right from the beginning, that everything outside conventional medicine is sheer quackery—and disastrous for the patient. Now that he knew otherwise, Bill tried to set aside his prejudices by adopting a new principle.

"I decided that a doctor should first try to treat his patient in a non-toxic way ... and only resort to drugs after all else had failed and there was no alternative."

Then one day a health food store owner got Bill interested in nutrition as a means of treating disease. He was excited. Here was a non-toxic means of healing that fit his guiding principle. While working at Kaiser and investigating chiropractic, he devoted his remaining time to the intense study of nutrition. Within a year he had become a lecturer in nutrition and vitamin therapy, and he had broadened his horizons to include the mysteries of herbal medicine.

At the same time he grew interested in the beneficial effects of meditation. For nearly three years he practiced a form of concentrated East Indian meditation in which he was taught to focus his mind, then refocus whenever it wandered. That improved his power of concentration and eventually led him to Da Free John, an enlightened western mystic who taught that "All is God," often using radical measures to prove to the members of his community that God was everywhere present.

In the meantime, Bill's studies of chiropractic, herbal medicine and nutrition began to turn sour.

"It wasn't long before I found the same fallacies in them that exist in standard medicine. They suppressed symptoms, were subject to fads and failed to treat the whole person. And there were no cohesive underlying principles, no holistic basis. So then I looked into acupuncture because it was an ancient system with definite principles that made sense."

He was seriously studying acupuncture when he happened to read a magazine article on homeopathy by William Gutman, MD, an elderly survivor from the days when the healing art still flourished at the turn of the century—before it was ambushed by the AMA and the drug companies. Curious, Bill hunted down the author and soon discovered that homeopathy was founded solidly on principles of incredible appeal.

"I was impressed that there were guiding principles and laws that dictated how medicines were prescribed. Standard medicine had nothing like that. Neither did nutrition or herbal medicine. I was highly intrigued."

Dr. Gutman told him of a one month's course—the only instruction on homeopathy then available—soon to be given in Millersville, Pennsylvania by the National Center for Homeopathy. This handful of clinicians, survivors of the purge, were now the leading homeopaths in America.

"So I took time off from Kaiser," Bill recalls. "and went back to Pennsylvania to take the course. Right from the beginning I was *really* impressed. Homeopathic theory was beautiful! The cure rate was remarkable. And the homeopaths I met were very experienced, extremely dedicated clinicians and fantastic people. They

65

had a very definite science behind them and they knew what they were doing. Unfortunately, they'd never had the benefit of good training."

For good reason. When the American Medical Assocation was formed in 1847, one of its expressed purposes was "... to stamp out the scourge of homeopathy." AMA members were forbidden to consult with or even associate with homeopaths. In fact one Connecticut physician was expelled from his local medical society for associating with a homeopath—his wife!

Nevertheless, by the turn of the century, one doctor out of five in America was a homeopath, and the numbers were steadily growing. Because homeopathy worked! It inexpensively produced real cures and was highly appealing to the public. But this strange branch of medicine was competing too effectively, cutting into allopathic profits. In 1911, in collusion with the drug companies, which were also losing profits, the AMA produced the Flexner Report which slandered homeopathy as out-dated, unscientific and a menace to the public. Using money and political muscle, the conspirators got the government to close down all but two homeopathic medical schools. Within a decade these too had folded.

So, by 1971—61 years later—Bill's teachers, the remnants of the earlier homeopathic community, had only informal training. They'd never had the benefits of the comprehensive curriculum and professional standards to be found in a homeopathic medical school.

"As much as I admired them," Bill says sadly, "they were unable to achieve the great results of the old masters. During the dark ages of homeopathy they heroically kept the art alive by reading and studying and teaching one another. My principal teacher, Dr. Maesimund Panos, was an inspiring example. Her husband and father had both been homeopaths."

Maesimund Panos

Mrs. Panos was an Ohio high school teacher, with children six and eight, when her husband, who had been the great hope of homeopathy, unexpectedly died of a heart attack in 1950. Determined to take his place, she quit her job, went to college in pre-med and, at the age of forty, was accepted into Ohio State University Medical School. She graduated, completed her internship, then trained as a full-fledged doctor under the best homeopaths of the time.

Finally, she began practice as a homeopath, working and studying and consulting with others to carry on the work of her late husband. Today, she's the Grande Dame of homeopathy, the matriarch of the art in this country, with a practice in Tipp City, Ohio.

Bill was impressed with "Maisie's" teaching and inspired by her dedication. After the course in Pennsylvania ended he asked her to take him on as an apprentice, something she'd never done before. Part of her mission in life was to hand the torch to bright young practitioners who might survive the dark ages and restore homeopathy to its rightful place. So she agreed. For a month, Bill accompanied her on her rounds, watching and listening and asking questions. "The more I saw," says Bill, "the surer I was that homeopathy was what I'd been searching for. But I wasn't sure I could learn it. It was just too complicated!"

But he decided to try. When he came back to work at Kaiser Hospital, Dr. Bill Gray, just turned thirty, dropped all his other interests and devoted himself exclusively to the study of homeopathy, working as hard as he could. Not long thereafter, an epidemic of Hong Kong Flu struck the San Francisco Bay Area. Thousands of people were deathly sick.

"At Kaiser," Bill remembers, "all we could offer them was 'bed rest, aspirin, fluids and wait two weeks.' It wasn't much help."

Then Bill began treating people homeopathically, using two remedies known to be effective for that particular epidemic, putting his new-found knowledge to work for the first time. He told his patients, "This may or may not help, but at least it can't hurt you, so let's give it a try."

To everyone's amazement, he completely cured 37 out of 40 cases—overnight! "That convinced me beyond any doubt that homeopathy worked."

Now Bill was ready to open a practice—but not as a homeopath. He wasn't ready for that. But he felt he could make a living, and "do more good than harm," by practicing nutrition, vitamin therapy and herbal medicine, along with a little chiropractic and homeopathy. And of course he wanted to deliver babies. So he quit his job at Kaiser and opened a small office in the little apple growing town of Sebastopol, sixty miles north of San Francisco.

Right from the start he called himself Bill Gray, not Dr. William Gray. And it wasn't because he was a glad-hander or back-slapper. That's not his personality at all. He explains, "I very consciously and deliberately call myself Bill to avoid erecting a barrier between myself and my patient. I never wear a white coat for the same reason. The word 'doctor' often separates the patient from the healer. I learned that in medical school, where they teach the strict separation of patient and doctor. Barriers and separation only make it harder to achieve the kind of openness and candid rapport that's essential in homeopathy between doctor and patient."

In his new practice Bill functioned mainly as a nutritionist. "I only did homeopathy when I felt competent," he explains. "At first I limited myself to acute prescribing, but gradually I got bolder and took a few chronic cases. I did a lot of home births, and before long I got in trouble. I let a midwife deliver a baby in a hospital labor room. They almost kicked me out of the hospital for that. But she'd delivered more babies than I had, and she was better at it than I was. Of course the local doctors couldn't see it that way. They put me on probation!"

Bill liked it in Sebastopol. "That was the happiest time in practice I ever had—because I was delivering babies." But the homeopathic part of his practice grew steadily as word spread of his success, and gradually nutrition, vitamin therapy and herbal medicine came to occupy less of his time. Homeopathy, he found, was far more effective than all the others combined! As he took on more and more chronic disease cases, the demands on his time and energy finally forced him to give up delivering babies.

"I hated to quit, but I just couldn't spend half the night somewhere out in the country, waiting for a baby to come. I had recently gotten married, and I didn't want to neglect my spiritual pursuits. But mostly it was the growing demands of my homeopathic practice. I was serious about it, and it took all the time I could give it."

Four years later, Bill was busier than ever practicing homeopathy. By now he had left Da Free John's commune, and he was no longer married. He was also growing progressively more frustrated with his inability to cure all his chronic patients.

"The old books described really miraculous cures in the deepest cases of a century ago, but I was only getting piddling results. I never saw the kind of miracles I read about. Obviously, I was doing something wrong."

He consulted with every good homeopath he could reach, but they weren't able to help. Then he got really dismayed when he realized that some of his patients were getting gradually worse.

"It was the same sort of thing I'd seen in nutrition. Their common symptoms were better, but overall—constitutionally—they were worse. I was beginning to sweat. Maybe I was doing more harm than good after all!"

Then he met George Vithoulkas, the world's foremost homeopath, in December, 1974. He had gone to a homeopathic conference in Washington D.C., looking desperately for help. With him he had brought detailed accounts of twenty cases that stumped him.

"What am I going to do with these?" he had asked George in a forum of young doctors like himself. George patiently listened and made some suggestions. Bill hurried home and followed the Greek physician's advice. Not surprisingly, a high percentage of his patients made dramatic recoveries. "Then I knew what I had to do—and where I had to do it."

He journeyed to Greece and spent a month following Vithoulkas around in his clinic in Athens. The local staff doctors took the master from room to room, presenting their cases and humbly asking for his advice. Bill accompanied them, eagerly observing, feverishly taking notes as Vithoulkas translated the discussion into English for his benefit.

"It was great!" he recalls, "I was really enthused. But when I went back to my practice in California, I quickly realized I was only a babe in the woods. I didn't know anything!"

The following year, Bill spent another month in Greece with Vithoulkas. Before it was over he knew he could never learn the art of homeopathy in just one month a year. He prevailed upon the master to take him on as an apprentice. Vithoulkas had never done

anything like that before, but he liked the young American's dedication and determination. So he agreed to teach him at the clinic
for three years. Delighted, Bill closed his practice in California.

"I just put everybody on hold while I went to Greece to learn
more about homeopathy."

Every day Bill went to the Athens clinic and accompanied
Vithoulkas on his rounds. But he also spent long hours alone with
the master. His education was divided into three phases: (1) homeopathic theory, (2) learning the symptom pictures of hundreds of
remedies and (3) homeopathic diagnosis, known as case analysis.
George's instruction in theory was rather unusual. It was Bill's job
to turn the master's tutorial lectures into books!

"George would free associate the contents of a chapter," Bill
explains, "then I would try to organize it and put it into good
English. George is more creative than systematic, so unscrambling
and reassembling what he told me was a very effective learning
process. By the time he was satisfied with what I'd written, I knew
the material backwards and forwards. By the time we were done,
we had written two books."

First came the introductory book, *Homeopathy: Medicine of
the New Man* (the blue book of chapter one), followed by the unex-
celled textbook, *The Science of Homeopathy* (part of which is condensed in chapter two).

Phase two—homeopathic remedies—meant solitary study
instead of lectures. For an average of sixteen hours every day, Bill
read and memorized the characteristics of all the major remedies
in a variety of books from George's library.

"My job was to grasp the underlying essence of each remedy
from the various accounts I found in different books, or from
George's descriptions on tape. I'd study a single remedy for hours
and days until I thought I really knew it. Then I'd go back to
George and try to explain what I thought the essense was. He'd listen, then he'd correct me. We kept working until I had it right."

Then Bill put the essences of the remedies into manuscipt
form, too. It was their fascinating accounts of Lycopodium (club
moss) and Natrum muriaticum (ordinary salt) in the brief Materia

Medica in *Medicine of the New Man* that so excited my interest in homeopathy. Most of the remedy essences Bill wrote about have not yet been published. They're still in first draft and have yet to be "worked up" to George's satisfaction.

The third phase of Bill's study, case analysis, was by far the most advanced—and difficult. It drew on both homeopathic theory and a knowledge of remedies, but depended even more on judgment and experience. "And experience was something I didn't have," Bill remembers. "George would take an actual case of his, written in Greek, and verbally translate it into English, while I furiously took notes. I'd take down the exact words the patient had said and all the nuances George had noted.

"Then I'd go home to my apartment and study the case. Somehow it never seemed to fit the knowledge I'd acquired. I'd bust my tail studying—all day and half the night. Then the next day I'd go back to George with the answer I'd worked out. All he'd say was, 'Nope, you're wrong.'

"So I'd go back home and study it again until this time I was pretty sure I had the right answer. Then I'd go back to him again and tell him what I thought. And all he'd say was, 'Nope.' So I'd go back and study it again. After three or four tries, depending on how compassionate he was feeling, he'd finally give me the answer. When he did, I'd say, 'Of *course*! Why didn't I see it!'"

Bill was given three or four cases every day, so the work soon began to pile up. Before long he was up to his eyes in unsolved Greek medical cases.

"In the beginning I failed almost a hundred percent of the time," Bill says, shaking his head in wonder. "It was all Greek to me for quite awhile. Then I began to understand that I couldn't be entirely intellectual all the time. I found out that, instead of building up a symptom picture, I needed to use a process of exclusion—sort of like a Hindu meditation. I learned to say to myself, 'It's not this, not that, not that, not that,' ruling out one remedy after another."

After a while, in self defense, he developed a kind of intuition that helped him quickly eliminate remedies that, in the end, couldn't fit the case. Gradually he gained the experience that helped him discriminate between almost identical sounding symptom pictures.

"What was weird is that a way of analyzing a case that worked on *one* set of symptoms would give me the wrong answer on another set that looked almost identical! It boggled my mind. I realized there was no way I could figure this out logically. Until I could gain enough experience, it seemed like I had to be intuitive or psychic!"

Bill had never worked so hard in his life. He drove himself relentlessly, studying, listening, questioning, writing. The apprenticeship with Vithoulkas had been scheduled for three years, but Bill worked so hard that he completed the agreed-upon agenda in two.

"It was the hardest work I ever did," he insists. "I went through Stanford Medical School and internship, but this was far harder than either one."

But it was wonderful training, the best any American homeopath had received for generations. Bill returned to California and reopened his practice, this time in the town of Fairfax, but he soon moved down to Berkeley to be in the center of the metropolitan San Francisco Bay Area. Almost immediately he began to teach what he had learned.

This was the beginning of his role as spokesman for America's homeopaths. It was more than coincidence that his return from Greece in 1978 also marked the beginning of the rebirth of homeopathy in America. He had justified the faith of Dr. Panos and her colleagues by bringing back the light that put an end to the dark ages. He launched the return to acceptability that homeopathy enjoys in the rest of the world, where it isn't being persecuted by a greedy orthodox medical establishment!

As soon as Bill returned he set up courses and went to work, training the staff in what is now Hahnemann Clinic. And in the next few years he trained another one hundred and fifty physicians across the country. Virtually every modern homeopath in America since the mid-seventies was trained, at least in part, by Dr. Bill Gray!

"I brought them to a certain point," he explains. "I took them as far as my limited capablities as a teacher permitted ... to a mediocre level. When I say 'mediocre,' I'm not just being modest. But I did the best I could."

Then he arranged for George Vithoulkas to come regularly to America for a month every year to give the advanced seminars that lifted his students to a higher more professional level. Some of these graduates have gone to Greece and served personal apprenticeships, similar to Bill's, with Vithoulkas. One of them, Roger Morrison of Hahnemann, is the most advanced of them all, Bill insists.

Roger Morrison

Roger had been a senior in medical school at the University of Tennessee when he happened to read an article by Bill in a magazine he picked up in a health food store. "I decided it was either a pack of lies or the greatest thing going," he remembers. "Right away I wrote Bill. When I didn't get an answer I wrote George Vithoulkas in Greece. Back came an invitation to attend a seminar on homeopathy."

His medical school refused to give him leave, but a friend in administration wangled permission. On arriving in Athens Roger went straight to the Athenian Clinic. The busy operation astounded him. Although thirty MD's were seeing patients in two buildings, the waiting room was packed. Each doctor spent forty minutes alone with a patient, then George would come in to review the case, consult and oversee the prescription. Fascinated, Roger watched and listened. When the waiting patients learned he was an American medical student, they crowded around to talk to him.

"In Greece," he explained, "American doctors are next to God. I had twenty beaming people telling me stories all at once of their miraculous homeopathic cures. They spoke mostly in Greek and sign language, but somehow I understood them. It was a powerful experience. After that I never thought of doing anything else. I had to be a homeopath. I already knew that allopathy didn't really cure anybody. And I'd gone into medicine to cure!"

By the time the seminar was over, Roger knew where he had

73

to come to learn. As soon as he returned home he began to study modern Greek and read everything he could find on homeopathy. "I could see it would be impossible to take cases in Greece without a knowledge of the language. And that's what I wanted to do. I didn't want to just watch. I wanted to work in George's clinic alongside his physicians."

In the meantime, along with other MD's, Roger took a one year course from Bill, spending one week every other month, plus a month in the fall with Vithoulkas. "That was electric. It was the first time homeopathy had been taught in this country as a science. When I was done I was eager to go to work—with Bill or George— but nothing worked out."

George was willing to take him into the Athenian Clinic on a Supervised Fellowship, but work permits for Americans were impossible to obtain. Finally he gave up and went to work in a hospital emergency room. Then one day George called to report that one of his patients, a powerful politician, had interceded. The coveted work permit had been granted. "I was astounded," said Roger. "It was the second time my homeopathic career had been rescued. I began to believe it was meant to be."

At first Roger stayed by the master's side, accompanying him on his rounds, night and day. His ability to converse in Greek was a great advantage. Later, he studied remedies and cases until his competency was proved to Vithoulkas' satisfaction. Finally he was given an office in the clinic and patients of his own. "After that, I learned mostly from the other doctors, some of whom had worked with George for 15 years. They still thought of themselves as his students."

After twenty-one months in Greece, Roger returned to America in 1984 and came straight to the Bay Area, where he helped merge five independent homeopathic practices into Hahnemann Family Clinic.

"He knows all the small remedies that I don't know," says Bill. "Here's a current example of Roger's expertise. I've been treating a psychotic woman for more than five years. In that time she's improved a great deal—but not for quite awhile. She seemed to be stuck. So yesterday I took her to Roger. I sat in while he took her case. His line of questioning brought out aspects of the case I hadn't suspected. It was brilliant! And it resulted in his prescribing a new remedy. I'm excited at her prospects!

"Roger has been able to go farther than the rest of us, because he's had so much more training. It's sort of a leapfrogging process. And it's bound to get even better now that we've got a medical school working again."

All that training—and more—is vital for a homeopathic physician who hopes to classically treat constitutional or chronic cases. To be truly effective, a high degree of training is essential. There isn't any shortcut. It takes dedication, time and energy to be what George calls, "consistent and reliable."

Bill amplifies what that phrase means. "You have to know when you've done harm ... as well as good. The professional must recognize when his remedy has created a disruption or a suppression. If you've given the wrong remedy, you need to know how to interpret the result—and what to do next. You even have to know when deliberately to suppress. All that's part of the job."

Homeopathy isn't foolproof. Far from it. Though highly dilute and non-toxic, the remedies act powerfully and can be dangerous to people with very weak vital forces, if prescribed incorrectly. The wrong remedy can wipe out certain people for years. Bill explains.

"I'm treating a woman who received two different remedies from another homeopath, spaced six weeks apart. They ruined her for ten years! They weren't really bad choices, but her doctor wasn't well enough trained to realize how weak her vital force was— -and prescribe accordingly. I'm still trying to bring her back.

"I make mistakes, too, all the time. But my training permits me to recognize the error *before* it can do any harm. Hopefully, I don't perpetuate the problem. That's the subtle, more sophisticated side of homeopathy. I emphasize it with my students: recognizing when you've made somebody better and when you've made them worse. The next step is to figure out what to do when you see you've made a mistake."

Thanks to Bill's ability to surmount the obstacles and go

beyond the limitations of his time, the homeopaths of the future will have a much easier time getting training—and acceptance. They won't need quite the dedication of the pioneers. And they'll probably be better homeopaths.

"Those who come after me," Bill says, "won't have to struggle like I did. They'll have a medical school to go to, and they'll probably be better homeopaths than I am. But to get good results they'll still need dedication. There's a direct correlation between the two. No doubt about it."

When Bill started practicing homeopathy back in 1971, northern California boasted only three old homeopaths who really weren't very good by modern standards—plus one lay prescriber and Bill. Bill helped organize a study group in the Bay Area so students could teach each other and consult.

"Bootstrapping," he calls it. "Our network attracted others in a typical Aquarian Conspiracy way. This group formed Hering Clinic in Berkeley while I was away in Greece."

The remaining homeopaths in the area soon joined Hering, making it the leading facility of its kind in the country. As a result, the Bay Area has become the bastion of classical homeopathy in America. A reorganization of Hering Clinic resulted in the creation of Hahnemann Clinic, which opened in January, 1985, just five months before I discovered it.

More than just a teaching clinic, Hahnemann became the nearest thing to a formal medical school in 1986, when thirty licensed health professionals from California and Oregon began a two-year course in classical homeopathy, devoting four full days a month to lectures and workshops while maintaining their regular practices. The faculty is headed by Bill and Roger and two others, aided by the rest of the Clinic's staff. George contributes when he's in residence, but isn't expected to be the primary force. His prize pupils are carrying the torch.

The International Foundation for Homeopathy in Seattle was the first teaching facility in the world to use videotapes of cured cases to show students what remedy pictures look like in the flesh. Hahnemann Clinic and George Vithoulkas have now followed suit.

Video is also perfect for showing diagnostic techniques. Bill explains.

"As the students watch the interview unfold, we stop it frequently to ask them, 'What remedy comes to mind?' And since we only use cured cases, they know that everything the patient on the tape says and does is a proven part of the picture of that remedy. They watch the homeopath doing the interview develop the threads that lead to the essence of the remedy. It's like watching a mystery unravel. It's a super way to teach. We've got over three hundred cured cases now on film in our library."

But television is no substitute for hard work and dedication. After training a hundred and fifty homeopaths, Bill has noted several patterns.

"The most promising applicants always express a deep dissatisfaction with other forms of healing. When they bitterly complain about their inability to cure their patients, we know they're dedicated ... not just looking for a new wrinkle. Or if they rave about *The Science of Homeopathy*, I know they're promising. Two or three times a week now we get calls from doctors who have read the book and 'couldn't put it down' and 'want to know more.' George's book makes a lot of converts."

George Vithoulkas

George Vithoulkas, ten years older than Bill, grew up in Greece during World War II. As a result of starvation and malnutrition, he developed chronic neck and back problems that kept him suffering terribly all through childhood and youth. He saw suffering all around him, and he wondered why humans should have to bear so much pain.

His contemplation of suffering seems somehow akin to Bill's yearning to enter the universe of others. Both provided motivation. George's search for understanding became a quest for spiritual enlightenment, and he studied all the spiritual literature he could find.

His aunt took care of him as a youth and saw to it that he attended the best schools and got the finest scientific education available. Largely by chance, young George Vithoulkas became a structural engineer, but his true goal in life was to make his way to India and find a guru who could aid his search for spiritual enlightenment. He went to South Africa to take a job that would permit him to save money for the trip to India. There he met a man who introduced him to homeopathy.

One day George's car broke down, stranding him for the weekend in a small town. He happened to have with him a copy of Boericke's Materia Medica with *Repertory*, a condensed encyclopedia of the characteristics of the principal homeopathic remedies. Having nothing better to do, George began reading it.

"It's like reading the phone book," Bill says. "It's really boring." But like many a man and woman before him—and since—George found there was something about homeopathy that tremendously excited and intrigued him.

As he read, he came to realize that this was what he'd been looking for. This was the answer, a way to relieve the worldwide suffering that so haunted him. Here was impeccable logic, scientific precision and impressive results. Forgetting about sleep, he devoured the homeopathic encyclopedia. Before the weekend was over, he'd read the big book cover to cover!

As soon as he could get to a bookstore, he intuitively picked out the very best books on homeopathy. For the next three and a half years he studied them religiously, sixteen hours a day, never taking a rest, devoting himself completely to the art that entranced him. There was nobody to teach him, no one at all. All he could do was read and read. Gradually he started treating friends and friends of friends. His method was exhaustive and exhausting. He would spend three full days on a case before prescribing.

Each day he would go back and interview his patient again and ask more questions, studying his notes half the night. But this devotion to detail paid off. Right from the start, the remedies he chose were correct and effective—almost a hundred per cent of the time! He was that strict, that dedicated. But he knew he badly needed formal training, too. So he finally made the long-planned trip to India.

He sought out gurus, as planned, but he also attended three different homeopathic medical colleges, the best India had to offer. He finally settled on one and went to work for his degree. It was soon discovered that he was far more advanced than the best professors. Before he was through he was teaching as well as studying—and treating the faculty and their families and friends homeopathically. In class, his professors often consulted him to confirm the accuracy of their teachings!

After graduation, Vithoulkas spent some time in Switzerland, treating Europe's elite, before returning to Greece in 1969. There he established the Athenian School of Homeopathy, a combination clinic and medical school.

One of his unique contributions to modern homeopathy is his comprehensive and intriguing "Definition of Health." Samuel Hahnemann, says Bill, didn't fully understand the concept. J.T. Kent came closer, but it remained for the Greek master to provide a precise definition that not only measures the health of the individual, but also shows how a patient progresses from ill health to cure.

"When I first heard it, it blew me away," Bill enthuses. "As a yardstick for measuring health, it's far better than any barrage of lab tests. It's a valuable tool for both professionals and patients because it provides a fresh prespective on how homeopathy heals holistically. I love it because it explains so much."

The Definition of Health—Expanded

As briefly noted in chapter two, health is measured homeopathically on three distinct levels or planes: the physical, the emotional and the mental. On the physical level, good health may be defined as freedom from the limitations of bodily symptoms and sensations. It's not the presence or absence of physical symptoms, it's the degree to which they affect one's consciousness and performance that measures physical health. It's freedom from having to place undue attention on your physical state. Bill elaborates:

"If your physical symptoms intrude on or occupy your attention, if they restrict your life, hamper you in any way or divide your attention, then they're afflicting your health. If you have a pain or an itch or a dryness or ache or paralysis or weakness of some sort that prevents you from fully focusing your attention, you have a physical disability. You're not completely healthy. To the extent that you have freedom from physical distractions, that's your particular degree of health."

On the emotional plane, health is freedom from being bound or controlled by your emotions and passions. Again, it's not the presence or absence of emotions, it's being free with them—rather than being controlled by them. It's the freedom to freely express the full range of emotions without being at their mercy. Bill explains:

"It's healthy to express emotions—as long as they're manageable and don't control your life. Truly healthy people—-emotionally—can fully express anxiety, jealousy, fear, joy, hate, lust, anger, ecstasy, etcetera—or they can set them aside in order to concentrate on the goal of the moment. These people aren't slaves to their passions. It's not whether you get irritable or depressed, the question is how does it affect you? Does the feeling become a mood, does it take you over, does it limit your performance? Or can you readily escape your passion and change your feelings? Good health is being free to choose and change."

On the mental plane, there are two tiers. The first is concerned with basic brain function: i.e. awareness of surroundings and memory of the past. Only the mentally disabled fail to qualify as healthy on this level. The second tier is the spiritual level, which has nothing whatever to do with religion. Health on this level is defined as "selfless creativity," a term that requires some explanation.

Bill says, " 'Selfless' doesn't mean being a martyr or sacrificing yourself for the happiness of others. On the contrary, self awareness and self-esteem are vital for good mental health. 'Selfless' in this context means being free to pay attention to the needs, aspirations and feelings of other people—as *well* as to yourself. It's neither selfishness nor the absence of self-concern. It's a sensitive mix of the two."

'Creativity' in George's definition uses the word in its broadest sense. The mentally healthy person is able to look at things in different ways, to synthesize from past experience, to display mental flexibility. And to work creatively and artisitically, using imagination and exhibiting curiosity.

"The mentally healthy person," says Bill, "can look at things anew, is open to new ideas, willing to reconsider, able to take a new slant on life."

So "selfless creativity" means that mentally healthy people are free to fully enjoy themselves. They are very aware of the feelings and needs of others, and work and play creatively for the benefit of both themselves and other people. That's true mental health.

Add to that the freedom to feel the full range of human emotions—without being controlled by any of them, and a physical state that does not limit or intrude on the rest of life ... and you have the homeopathic definition of health, as devised by George Vithoulkas. Good health then is true freedom! And true freedom means happiness. "Show me a man who's truly healthy, and I'll show you a happy man!"

This ideal state of health is the homeopath's goal for his patient. And it's the yardstick he's constantly applying as he sensitively watches and listens to his patient. It's the norm that defines symptoms. Every expression of the patient is judged against this yardstick, from the first moment he walks in the door until the cure is finally complete. The homeopath must constantly ask him or herself, while cataloging and delineating the patient's every symptom, "Is that a limitation of freedom, or not?"

George's definition is also used constantly to measure progress toward a cure and reversals and suppressions. The appearance or disappearance of symptoms, homeopaths know, generally takes place in an unvarying order. Genuine cure proceeds from above downward and from inward outward, and, more importantly, from the deeper to the superficial. This is profoundly important to the homeopath. The mental plane is deepest. The emotional plane is in between, and the physical plane is most superficial.

So, from the homeopath's viewpoint, if the emotional plane is still disturbed but the mental plane has cleared after a period of treatment, a cure is taking place. Or if physical symptoms remain but the emotional plane has cleared, progress is being made. And when skin irritations remain but the deeper organs are healed, the cure is proceeding. And the opposite progression is just as revealing. Bill explains:

"If the remedy I give improves your skin rash but you become depressed or lose your energy or creativity, that tells me a suppression has taken place instead of a cure. Then I know the remedy was wrong. So now I must reconsider your case or gather more data in order to find the remedy that will cure your entire being. I rely absolutely on George's definition of health to both diagnose the patient and tell me how I'm doing."

Even before Hahnemann College of Homeopathic Medicine opened in 1986, Bill was incredibly busy in his dual role as full time practitioner—and full time administrator, spokesman, promoter, politician and teacher. Consider his activities the week of our October conference on my way to Hawaii. After a full day's caseload on Monday, he spent all evening at a meeting.

"On Tuesday," he recalls, "I had a severe AIDS case—a 46-year-old man who's going to die in six months if I don't do something. He was here two and a half hours—all the way through my lunch hour. And when he finally left, the patient he'd displaced was still there waiting. So I got nine minutes for lunch!"

Bill was just getting started on his afternoon appointment schedule when the police brought in a man who had just walked out of a nearby hospital with manic depressive psychosis. He refused to see anyone but Bill. So Bill had to squeeze the man into an already full schedule. After making his evening phone calls to patients, Bill managed to get home and fall in bed at six-thirty. The next thing he knew it was the following morning and his alarm clock was ringing. He had slept thirteen hours straight!

Wednesday was another big day.

"Besides my local patients, I had a man fly in from Los Angeles. He had suicidal depression to the point where he could easily kill himself. I couldn't safely make him wait. Then an executive with a fatal disease arrived from Cincinnati, hoping for help. He'll die in three years if I can't cure him. So I had to struggle through those two extra cases."

It was six thirty when he finished his evening calls and stretched out on his office couch to read sixty-odd pages of my maunscript. Afterward, he attended a staff meeting that ran until midnight, so it was one in the morning before he got to bed. On Thursday his morning was jammed, but he did get to read *Newsweek* for a few minutes while he ate lunch. And when his caseload was finally over for the day, he had to return patient's phone calls, then attend a workshop in the library on some little known remedies Roger had brought back from Greece.

When Bill gets a chance to relax, he likes to read, but that doesn't happen very often. After I innocently mentioned several books I thought he'd like, he pointedly said "I don't read, I work!"

But one Sunday afternoon, browsing in a bookstore, he found a copy of *Yaeger* and bought it. He was absolutely committed to completing a pile of back paperwork that afternoon, but he decided he'd read just one chapter ... to get the flavor of it. "Well, I couldn't put it down. I forgot all about the work and read all afternoon and half the night ... and most of Monday night, too, until I finished it. But that kind of thing keeps me human. If there was nothing in my life but homeopathy, I'd go nuts."

Right now Bill's single purpose in life is to firmly establish Hahnemann College of Homeopathy. "It's hard," he says, "to exaggerate what a tremendous thing it is to open a homeopathic medical school again—after three quarters of a century of darkness. Because this is the school that's going to train all the homeopaths that will treat all those sick people out there in the hinterlands. That's how I see it. When I look back on my life, I expect to see that this was the purpose for doing what I did."

Now that the job is nearing completion, Bill hopes to make up for lost time.

"There's still time for me to go out and live like a normal human being. I'm young enough. I'd like to get married again and have kids, do all the normal things I've missed. And my latest passion is gliding. I guess I get it from my father. I'm just learning, but I love it. It's very peaceful up there, soaring among the clouds ... very different from homeopathy! When I'm up there in the sky, I can forget for awhile that anyone is sick."

5

Trouble in Paradise

Battling Tropical Fungus ... A Tough Decision ... My Vital
Force Survives A Test ... Deanne Becomes A Home
Prescriber ... I Undergo A Personality Change

We arrived in Hawaii in November and drove to our house through
torrential rain. A hurricane had narrowly missed the island, bringing stifling heat and incredible humidity. That night I felt like I was
sleeping in a sauna, breathing liquid air. The rain had stopped but
the trees were dripping, and so was I. The temperature and
humidity were close to a hundred, and my thick mountain blood
was boiling.

In the morning, not surprisingly, my crotch rash was much
worse. I washed, powdered myself with Tinactin, put on shorts and
hoped the ventilation would help. The next day my crotch was
worse and I began to walk bowlegged to avoid the soreness and
itching. And my brow, which had only been mildly chapped when I
arrived, suddenly turned red and swollen. Clearly, the climate
change was overwhelming my defenses, so I called Bill.

"Frankly, I'm not surprised," he said blandly. "That's why I
wanted to suppress your crotch rash. There's just too much mold
and fungi over there. I figured your rash would go crazy. It's just
too much stress for your vital force to handle all at once."

"Why didn't you tell me beforehand?"

"Because I didn't want you to cancel your trip."

"But I can't *handle* this!" I protested. "What do I do? Where do I go?" As I waited the options flashed before me. Echo was closed and freezing. Walker was still toxic with pollen. Now Hawaii was overloaded with fungus.

"It's going to be all right," he soothed. "Believe me, I don't want you to suffer. We'll just have to treat you allopathically.

"What does *that* mean?" I asked suspiciously.

"I want you to see a good dermatologist.... Of course his drugs will antidote your remedy."

"Antidote?" I was shocked. "Can't you treat this homeopathically? What about acute remedies?"

"For what you've got they're much too mild and slow. Especially in Hawaii." His tone turned sympathetic. "Listen, Bob, life goes on. I don't want you to change your lifestyle just to stay on the cure. You're not that sick."

"The drugs I need would really antidote my remedy?" I had to be sure. The gains I'd made were too precious to give up.

"I'm afraid so. Some people with strong vital forces get away with it, but ninety percent of the time it stops the process."

"For how long?"

"Maybe three or four months. Look, it's no big deal, no ultimate disaster. It won't hurt to suppress for awhile. Find a competent dermatologist and try to get a precise diagnosis along with your prescription. Then call me. If his prescription sounds reasonable, I'll probably let you take it."

Within two minutes of my arrival in the dermatologist's office, he was already writing prescriptions! He gave me Prednisone for my allergies, Cloxacillin antibiotic for the infection and Trideselin ointment for my rashes—enough to last for a week. As he started to leave, I asked, "What do you think I've got?"

"Allergy with bacterial staph infection."

"What can I expect?"

"Substantial improvement within forty-eight hours." He left and a nurse brought the bill.

Bill was out to lunch when I called and wouldn't be back until two pm. It was now only ten. It was going to be a long four hours. My crotch looked like hamburger and I walked like a man who'd messed his pants. I was frightened by the speed with which the

85

crust was spreading from my brow toward my eyes. At last it was time to call. As I started to dial it hit me. I had forgotten the three hour time differential! I had missed my phone date and it was now nearly five. The switchboard would be closing any moment. When I hastily called Karen she told me Bill was with a patient, but she'd try to get him to call me when he was through. I said I'd wait.

It was easily ninety degrees in the shade and my clothes were plastered to my body. When people approached my phone, I told them I was waiting for a call from my doctor. A glance at my face sent them scurrying. When Bill finally called I reported the dermatologist's diagnosis and prescription.

"Don't take *any* of it," Bill said tersely.

"But what's the alternative?"

"There isn't any."

"But what *else* can I do?" I wailed. I can't go *on* like this!" I knew I sounded half hysterical, but I didn't care.

There was a pause. "Okay, Bob," he said kindly. "I think I get the picture now. I'm afraid the phone's a poor vehicle for judging desperation. Take it and we'll pick up the pieces later. If it gets worse by the hour, you don't have much choice. I want you to enjoy yourself."

I hobbled into the drugstore with mixed feelings. I was hungry for relief but saddened by the need to kill the remedy that had been working for me now for four months. I hated what I was doing, but I had to escape my misery. So I took the drugs, fervently hoping I wouldn't lose all my gains.

The following morning I was fifty percent better, and the morning after that the yellow scabs were gone from my brow and my crotch had faded to a tender pink. Talk about wonder drugs! It wasn't hard to understand how magic like this made people forget about side effects, especially those that came later or couldn't be seen! To Deanne's dismay, I cut my drug dosage in half. I knew that all the suppressive medicine I ingested now would ultimately have to be expelled by my vital force, a process that might take months.

After three days my crotch and brow were nearly normal. Whatever had attacked me seemed stone cold dead, so I quit the drugs altogether. If symptoms returned I could always start popping pills again.

Thus ended my first eventful week in paradise!

Lying on the beach a few days later alone, I decided I couldn't have done differently. I'd simply had to have relief. I was lucky to get it so quickly. I wondered when Bill would let me start over. It was hard to imagine him mailing me more Tuberculinum without a thorough diagnosis, and I knew he hated to prescibe on the phone. It looked like I'd have to forget homeopathy for awhile.

Too bad! My benefits had been significant. Deanne had recently remarked, "I've never seen your forehead look so good. It always used to be so red." And it wasn't hypersensitive to sunburn any more. But what pleased me most was my freedom from heartburn. I used to live on Rolaids. Now they were no longer a part of my life.

I was reminded of a story Dr. Nelson, the San Francisco chiropractic internist, liked to tell about how we adjust to change. An elderly Scotsman had come to him on crutches with agonizing lower back pains. After a month of treatment the old man started coming on just one crutch. Another month and he was able to hobble in without crutches. But a month later he announced that he wouldn't be coming any more.

Fearing the old man had financial problems, Dr. Nelson asked why. The Scotsman looked at him in surprise. "Why, because ye haven't helped me, a course!" he said reprovingly. "Me back still hurts!" The man honestly could not see the progress he'd made until he was reminded that he was free of his crutches. It had happened too slowly. All he knew was that his back still hurt.

Exactly one week, almost to the hour, after I popped the last Prednisone, I stepped out of the shower and discovered to my horror that several red welts had returned to my crotch. "Oh, *no!*" I groaned. "Not again!" Was infection unavoidable? Must I live on drugs? Did I quit too soon? I couldn't stand the thought of going through it all again.

The next morning the itch in my left ear and toe had returned. So had the welts on my elbow. The pattern seemed vaguely familiar. Of course! This was the exact set of symptoms I'd brought with me from the mainland. Only the roughness on my brow was missing. Since these were proven Tuberculinum symptoms, perhaps my vital force had survived! I cautioned myself against getting too excited.

The next day my brow began to roughen and redden. I never thought I'd be so pleased to see a rash. The evidence now seemed conclusive. My vital force was alive and back at work. At first it seemed a miracle. But after further deliberation, I decided it wasn't. Bill had said drugs stop the process ninety percent of the time. But he'd also rated my vital force at nine on a scale of ten. So it seemed a 90%–90% standoff. Statisticians might disagree, but to me that meant my vital force had had a 50–50 chance of surviving all along.

Whatever the explanation, I was delighted. Then, six days later, the rash in my crotch began to redden and spread. This wasn't the Tuberculinum. The dreaded infection was back! At the dermatologist's suggestion, I bought Micatin and prayerfully applied it, but the rash grew steadily worse. By the time I gave up and went to see him again, both my crotch and the crust on my brow were as bad as before.

"It's the Staph again," he snapped. "Can't you manage to keep yourself clean? My prescription is the same but this time you bet-ter take it for a week. In fact, ten days would be better."

After two days on drugs my crotch and brow were once again clear. Getting well wasn't the problem. It was staying that way in Hawaii without drugs. This time when I quit I invoked a program of rigorous hygiene. Deanne snatched everything I might have infected and threw it in the washer: clothes, sheets, towels, even paint rags. For my part, I scrubbed vigorously three times a day, and tried to forget my past afflictions.

To celebrate we went to the beach where I promptly got sun-burned. That night my face was red and hot. I remembered that Aloe was wonderful for sunburn, and it was growing wild in our garden. I sliced off a chunk and rubbed the clear slime on my face. Relief was immediate and lasting. Aloe wasn't homeopathic, but it was natural and it worked. A week later I got sunburned again. But this time the Aloe didn't help. Instead of relief it brought redness and itching. The reaction was vaguely familiar. Then I remembered

Deanne's moisturing cream ... and before that the Vaseline. If my vital force was rejecting the Aloe, it must still be alive!

Sure enough, eighteen days after my second round of drugs, all my Tuberculinum symptoms came roaring back at once. It felt like a family reunion. My vital force had survived after all! Once again the antibiotics had somehow wiped out the infection without antidoting the Tuberculinum. Deanne was not amused, and my feelings were mixed. I was pleased, of course, that the remedy was still working, but I couldn't face the prospect of another crippling round of infection. My poor skin was worn out—and so was the rest of me. My vital force might be triumphant, but I felt like a fighter feebly hanging on the ropes.

A month passed with no return of the devastating infection that had twice sent me whimpering to the dermatologist for antibiotics. Frequent vigorous washing seemed to be the answer, though the cooling weather may have helped. And my body might have built some defenses.

Then a new and mysterious ailment beset me. While lifting heavy tree trunks and rocks in the yard, I managed to hurt my left shoulder and back. When the job was done, my back got worse instead of better! A husband and wife team of holistic chiropractors made repeated adjustments, but the relief didn't last. The pains returned soon after each adjustment. The Tuberculinum, they insisted, was to blame. It was possible. I'd once had chronic back pains of just this sort. Deanne thought they might be a "return of old symptoms". I'd have to ask Bill.

Meanwhile, Deanne discovered that a local naturopath named Michael Traub was beginning a series of workshops on homeopathic first aid and home prescribing. She had long been eager to get a homeopathic kit for family use. When she found that Dr. Traub had studied with Bill Gray, she was hooked. So we drove the 60 miles down the island's west coast for the first workshop.

Michael Traub turned out to be a slim, softspoken young man with a boyish smile ... and a strong resemblence to Samuel Hahnemann! He began by candidly telling us how he found his way to homeopathy. With an allopathic dermatologist for a father and a nurse for a mother, he had always planned to be a doctor. But after completing a pre-med course in college, he couldn't get into medical school.

"It was a shock to be turned down. I felt rejected," he admitted. "I'd never considered doing anything else, except counseling. Now I had to look for alternatives."

Casting about, he answered an ad that offered a homeopathic cure for pollen allergies. He'd long been plagued by severe hayfever. Shots hadn't helped and he hated the side effects he got from antihistamines. To his amazement, the homeopathic remedy brought great and immediate relief. The homeopath told him of a naturopathic college in Portland, Oregon, that offered instruction in a variety of natural, non-toxic holistic therapies ... including homeopathy. He promptly applied and was accepted.

"My dad was really upset," he admitted. "He told me I was crazy and wasting my time. But it sounded like just what I was looking for. When I read George Vithoulkas's *The Science of Homeopathy*, I knew I'd made the right choice."

After graduation and four years of practice in damp, chilly Portland—consulting from time to time with Bill Gray—-young Dr. Traub moved to Hawaii to set up his own practice. He came partly because the island state is one of only nine that recognizes naturopaths—and partly to get warm.

After the lecture I urged Deanne to tell him about her fruitless attempts to get rid of a persistent cough and sore throat. When she did and asked to make an appointment, he said, "What about right now?" and waved us into his office.

After establishing Deanne's basic symptoms, he asked about her sleeping habits, appetite and moods. Then he tried to discover the precise character of her cough by a barrage of questions about what made it better or worse, critical times of day, her response to heat and cold, sleeping and waking, drinking and eating, etc. He felt her forehead for fever and examined her tongue closely. "I think Rumex should do the job," he said at last and gave her a vial of pellets.

With Deanne taken care of, he asked me about my case and Bill Gray. I gave him a brief account of my adventures.

"Your face looks awfully dry," he said frowning.

"It is," I admitted, "but I'm not supposed to use anything to keep it moist . . . like Vaseline."

"Bill Gray might not approve," he said, smiling mischievously, "but I've got something I'd like to give you. It's called Calendula, a homeopathic lotion made from French Marigolds. It's better than vaseline and so mild that almost no one reacts to it."

"You wouldn't consider it suppressive?"

"Not at all."

"Then I'm ready to try it. I'm tired of skin that feels like parchment."

He produced a vial of yellow salve, and I rubbed some into my forehead. Relief was immediate and delicious. After using it for several days my face was comfortable and soft again. Then I quit. I didn't want a repetition of the violent reactions I'd had to Aloe, Vaseline and Deanne's moisturizing cream. But it was good to know relief was waiting if I needed it.

In response to a letter from Bill, I wrote about changes I'd been experiencing. "I'm breathing through my nose more than ever before in my life . . . in spite of humidity that I've always associated with greater congestion. Sometimes I just stop what I'm doing to enjoy the easy passage of air through my nose. Being able to breathe better is a big factor in my reduced irritability. . . . You warn that, even though my Tuberculinum symptoms are back, my vital force may not be working quite well enough to actually heal. But I'm not worried. I feel so much better I'm convinced that it's taking me toward a cure. . . ."

At Michael Traub's next workshop, Deanne told him the Rumex had stopped her cough and sore throat. And she bought his inexpensive 30-remedy treatment kit, along with the companion books he recommended, *Everybody's Guide to Homeopathic Medicines*, a yellow paperback by Cummings and Ullman, and *Homeopathic Medicine at Home* by Panos and Hemlich.

I was glad to have the kit and the introduction to its contents, but I was skeptical about how much we'd use it. Our little family, it seemed to me, was rarely sick or hurt. But here's what happened in the next three weeks. . . .

One night after dinner, while reading on the couch, I was suddenly seized with excruciating stomach cramps. Writhing and groaning on the floor, I tried to massage what I imagined to be a kinked intestine—without success. Doctor Deanne was soon standing over me, firing questions as she thumbed through *Everybody's Guide.* . . .

I just wanted to be left alone to my misery, but she merely cataloged that desire as one of my symptoms!

"Colocynthis would be perfect for cramping clutching abdominal pains," she said briskly, "but it's not in the kit. Have you recently experienced anger or an insult to your sense of injustice?"

It was possible, I admitted. I *had* been angry at dinner.

"Then the best remedy we've got is Mag phos," she decided, using the homeopathic shorthand for Magnesium phosphorica, phosphate of magnesia. She picked a tiny vial from her kit and shook four tiny sugar pellets into the cap. "Open your mouth, tilt back your head and lift up your tongue," she commanded.

I did as I was told, and she deftly dropped the pellets under my tongue. Then I caught my breath and braced for another wave of cramps. It came but was substantially weaker. After one last mild spasm, the agonizing pain in my stomach disappeared.

A few days later, Deanne burned her finger on a hot pan while cooking. She immediately stuck her finger in ice water while she leafed through the yellow book. The indicated treatment was the same Calendula cream that Michael had given me for my face. It worked as well for Deanne as it had for me. The pain was entirely gone in half an hour.

A week later she deeply cut a finger while slicing a roast. Once the wound was closed and dry, a coating of Calendula promoted rapid healing.

Our six-year-old daughter, Gellie, came home crying one afternoon. A boy had dropped a brick on her big toe. The skin wasn't broken but the pain was intense. Deanne riffled through the notes she had made in class, checked in the yellow book and decided on Arnica. It was excellent, Michael had told us, for immediate treatment of pain and shock. Deanne gave Gellie a dose and wiped away her tears, but half an hour later the toe still hurt. At our next workshop, Deanne asked Michael why the Arnica hadn't helped.

"Because it wasn't quite the right remedy. Hypericum—which we haven't discussed yet—happens to be specific for smashed fingers or toes—anyplace where there are lots of nerve endings."

One evening I complained that my ankles were itching madly, but I couldn't see any bites or rash. Deanne took a look, found a series of tiny white bumps, and decided it was "something like nettles," since we had hiked that afternoon through stiff dry grass that had chafed our ankles.

She made me try both hot and cold compresses to see which felt better. Having ascertained that the itching was "worse wtih heat," she gave me a dose of Apis (bee venom). The next day the itching was gone. In the space of just three weeks, Dr. Deanne had turned into a formidable home prescriber, and her kit had already paid for itself.

Sitting on the beach with Deanne one afternoon, I told her, somewhat hesitantly "I seem to be undergoing a personality change.

"Really?" She sounded mystified. "What's changed?"

"Some of my Tuberculinum keynotes."

"Well, you can't change your dad's TB, but I *have* noticed that you don't chase cats anymore. In fact now you talk to them and let them rub up against your legs. I'll be darned! That *is* quite a change! And yesterday when I offered to cook you bacon for lunch you weren't interested."

Her eyes narrowed. "How do you feel about pine trees?"

"I don't know. It's been six months since I saw one. But I haven't been pining for them either. . . ." She groaned.

Bill had told me last October that I'd feel better overall—not just physically—this winter in Hawaii. Now I was beginning to see what he meant. I was happier, more content, more vital and alive. Mentally, I'd gotten more accomplished than I expected. There was a decided upward trend in my laughter/anger ratio. And maybe I was a touch more tolerant and patient than I had been. It made me wonder what came next?

In April a storm rocked the islands for weeks, bringing drizzle and clouds. Before long Deanne began to cough. "My sore throat is back, and the Rumex doesn't help," she complained. "It happens every time there's a change in the weather ... or climate. I'm getting sick of it!"

"Sounds like a chronic condition. Since we change climates three times a year, maybe you should get a constitutional from Bill when we get back?"

"I guess I better."

When it came time in mid April to pack up and fly back to the mainland, I found the procedure was far less stressful than before. Waiting had always annoyed me. But our long, three flight day, with all the waiting in airports, now seemed no more taxing than a stroll down the beach.

6

Four Converted Young Docs

Linda Johnston MD ... Matt Vuksinich MD ...
Vicky Menear MD ... and Mark Rosen DO

Heralding an end to the dark ages of homeopathy, Hahnemann Clinic opened the first homeopathic medical school in America in over 60 years, in 1986. Bill introduced me to four of his ex-students, all in their mid thirties. Each has a different situation and background, but all are dedicated to the healing art they so recently have discovered ... and willing to pass up the lifestyle and riches that allopathy could have given them for the satisfaction of actually curing their patients. All these young converts were proud members of Hahnemann College of Homeopathic Medicine's first graduating class in the summer of 1988.

Linda Johnston, M.D., a petite general practitioner operating in Van Nuys (Los Angeles), has incorporated homeopathy into what used to be a purely allopathic practice. The graduate of the University of Washington completed her studies in 1980 and opened an office a year later. But after two years she began to grow dissatisfied with the tools and skills at her disposal.

"I wanted to do more," she explained, "so I began to investigate how different cultures, past and present, solved their health care problems. I was looking for wisdom I could glean and apply." Then one day in September, 1985, Linda happened to bump her knee on the corner of her coffee table. A friend—and homeopathic lay prescriber—happened to be there and offered her a dose of Arnica.

"The little sugar pellets were so small," she remembered, smiling, "I didn't think they could hurt me, so I took them. I bruise easily and I expected to wear a black and blue kneecap for weeks. I also expected lasting pain. But in five hours I had a pair of matching kneecaps and the pain was entirely gone. I was amazed!

"That experience made me think. If what had happened to me was real, then a lot of what I knew about healing wasn't true! Should I believe what happened or stick with what I knew? I decided to believe what had happened. From that moment on I considered myself a homeopath. I didn't have any training, but at heart I was a homeopath."

Linda was grateful for the first-hand experience. "I don't think I would have believed my case if I had read about it in a book. It would sound too miraculous. But I couldn't deny my personal experience." After sifting the wisdom of the ages in books, Linda had found what she'd been searching for . . . in her own living room!

"Unlike a lot of what I'd been studying in other cultures, it had a scientific basis. It didn't depend on faith healing or chanting or spiritual energy or secret concoctions. It was structured and meticulous and free of exceptions. It was just what I'd been hoping to find." Within three months Dr. Johnston was taking the IFH post graduate course in homeopathy in Seattle. Then she began cautiously incorporating elements of homeopathy into her traditional Los Angeles general medical practice.

"It's been a slow transition, medically and economically, but extremely rewarding and exciting! Everywhere I go I find myself talking homeopathy. Sit next to me on an airplane and you're going to be exposed to it! But I still believe the best introduction is to personally experience the incredible curing effects of an acute remedy . . . the way I did. Homeopathy's just too hard to explain, and it sounds too good to be true. Sometimes I feel like a nut on a soap box when I pour out anecdotes to someone who's never heard of it."

Unlike many doctors, Linda believes people should learn to

treat themselves. "I think everybody should become a lay homeo-pathic prescriber. It's so easy to use the little first aid kid for treat-ing acute conditions. Then you know the miracle for yourself. I think that's the best way to promote homeopathy."

Linda provided me with the three page tract she wrote to introduce homeopathy to her allopathically oriented patients. I complimented her on the apt analogies that helped make the sub-ject comprehensible. She smiled. "I use analogies a lot in my prac-tice. Initially, I try to make an assessment of the patient in terms of education and interests, as well as symptoms. Then I make per-sonal analogies involving their bodies, their symptoms and home-opathy. It helps me communicate better."

But not all her patients are ready for homeopathy. "Some peo-ple would leave and go someplace else if I insisted on treating them homeopathically," she explained. "I'm a healer first and a homeopath second. Sometimes I feel a little schizophrenic giving allopathic drugs because I know I'm hurting the patient while get-ting rid of his symptoms. That bothered me a lot until I realized that's the best I can do for some people. I believe drugs are a lot safer in a homeopath's hands than in the hands of most allopaths."

Homeopathy is just part of Linda's practice, but the demand is rapidly growing. Her day begins with constitutional homeopathic cases. Then she switches to traditional practice, where she fre-quently uses homeopathic remedies to treat acute conditions. I bluntly asked her if she felt competent to do constitutional prescribing.

"I'm just a beginner," she admitted, "but the best way to learn it is to do it. It was scary at first to take constitutional cases, but I decided that the longer I waited the harder it would get. I try to compensate for my inexperience and lack of training by fully informing my patients and giving them extra good care. Homeo-paths are so open and friendly that I've always been able to get help on tough cases. There isn't the competitiveness and secrecy and pride that I see among allopaths. I keep working until I'm sure I've got the whole remedy picture. And I often consult with Bill."

Linda limits her new constitutional patients to three a week to make sure she has all the time she needs.

"Some of my cases are extremely difficult—people who've been everywhere and tried everything to get relief. Others are easy to diagnose, and the remedy picture is soon clear. Either way, my integrity demands that I give each case all my skill and attention. Sometimes I'm up half the night studying a tough case. As I learn more and get better, I'll probably get faster and be able to do more. My goal right now is to perfect my skills as much as possible—not to build a big homeopathic practice."

As soon as she completed the IFH course, Linda began the two year course at Hahnemann College. She also signed up for all of George Vithoulkas's seminars in this country, and she's been going abroad for further study, taking courses worldwide. "Since I'm devoting my medical attention to homeopathy," she explained, "I want all the instruction I can get."

Personable Matthew Vuksinich, M.D., put himself through Northwestern University's medical school by working as a wandering troubador with his brother, playing the mandolin in the restaurants of San Francisco's North Beach. Halfway through his residency as a surgeon he began to grow disillusioned with conventional medicine. When he was done he took a job in the Emergency Room of Kaiser Hospital in San Francisco ... to postpone a decison on his future.

"After all those tough years in medicine, I didn't want to start over. I thought I'd work ER (Emergency Room) for maybe a year, then make myself go back to surgery, but I stayed and stayed, and pretty soon I realized I was only there for the paycheck." After three years at Kaiser, Matt was bitter about wasting his life in medicine. He wished he'd stayed with the mandolin and become a musician.

"I was just about ready to quit medicine, and was seriously exploring what to do with the rest of my life, when by accident I stumbled onto homeopathy. The timing was perfect." A friend's wife was suffering from a breast abscess, described to Matt as a big red fluctuant tender mass. She went to Hahnemann Clinic where a single highly dilute dose of Belladonna cured her completely in just a few hours!

"I still remember the story she told me. About two hours after taking the Belladonna she got really sick. Her temperature shot up from 102 to 104. She started vomiting and soon fell asleep. When she woke up three hours later, the damn thing was gone. She was cured! I couldn't believe it. As far as I was concerned, Belladonna was a poison! All I knew about homeopathy at the time was the med school joke about medicine so weak there wasn't anything there!"

But Matt had reason to know the cure was extraordinary. His own wife had been afflicted with the same sort of abscess just six months before. He had given her massive doses of Tetracycline and Erythromycin and several other powerful drugs ... three times a day for two weeks. It was the standard approach and all he knew at the time. But the infection kept recurring and wasn't obliterated until she had suffered four long painful relapses. Clearly, allopathic wonder drugs hadn't matched the miracle of Belladonna!

A few months later, his friend's wife again took her little girl to Hahnemann, this time with a bad earache. "These guys gave her some weak remedy and within an hour she was totally asymptomatic. We always treated earache with massive doses of antibiotics, but we never came close to results like that!"

Curious, Matt wrote Hahnemann and learned about its various courses. "I went to one of the Wednesday night workshops, just to see what these flakes looked like. But they didn't seem like flakes, so when George Vithoulkas came to town I went to one of his sessions. After all, he was supposed to be the best. What he said went completely over my head, but the audience and the questions impressed me. It didn't sound like space cadet medicine to me."

Matt wanted to know more, so he read Hahnemann's *Organon* and Kent's lectures. That did it. "Suddenly I was sold. I just knew what I was reading was utterly true. It was an approach to healing that I'd never even dreamed of, but it struck some kind of chord. After that I was a homeopathic junkie. And the timing was exquisite. I had been ready to go broke rather than stay with allopathic medicine. Now I knew exactly what to do."

But it wasn't to be easy. Matt's wife had left him with two young children to raise. He had to continue working in various emergency rooms to pay the bills while he studied homeopathy. But now he had a goal and a new perspective.

"In retrospect I saw how ineffective our ER treatment had been. Kids who had originally come in with eczema came back four months later with earache. Then three months after that they were back with sore throat, then bronchitis and after three years they had asthma. The pattern and progression were well marked. We weren't helping *any*body. We didn't know it, of course, but our drugs were merely suppressing. To us, these were just allergic kids. We didn't know our drugs were making them sicker!"

But that's all behind him now. Matt's long-range dream is a homeopathic practice somewhere out in the country. But short range he planned to open a small practice, hoping in a few years to gain enough experience to beg for a job in the Clinic. To his shock and delight, the Clinic offered him a job when he graduated. "I was flattered and ecstatic. It's wonderful to be doing something I believe in, something I really want to do. After wishing for years that I hadn't become a doctor, it's great to find out that my time wasn't wasted. I just hope I can learn to do it right."

Vicky Menear, MD, a tan athletic-looking lady with a blond pony-tail, attended classes at Hahnemann College in shorts and a baggy sweatshirt inscribed, "Hugs are Good Medicine!" During her fourth year of medical school in Pennsylvania she was diagnosed as having multiple sclerosis. That was long before she'd heard of homeopathy. "At the time, there didn't seem much I could do about it," she shrugged. "I just slept a lot, changed my diet and tried to maintain."

By the time she finished her internship she was disgusted with allopathic medicine and decided to forget about healing for awhile. It wasn't easy. Helping people get well was what she wanted to do. In medical school she had been criticized by her professors for being too close to her patients and too open with them. "Getting close helped me understand them," she explained. "You have to understand the problem before you can help."

Shortly after quitting medicine, while in England with her husband, she took a three week lecture course in homeopathy—

mainly out of curiosity. "It felt good to me," she said, "like a drink of cold water when you're dying of thirst. I felt like I'd wasted all those years studying medicine."

Back in the U.S., at the suggestion of noted homeopath Henry Williams, she took the National Center for Homeopathy's three week course, receiving instruction from Bill Gray, Ben Hole, Richard Pitcairn and Catherine Coulter, among others. And she read voraciously: Kent, Hahnemann, Clark, Boericke and others. Vicky was reluctant to start practicing with so little training but Williams insisted. "You'll do fine in homeopathy because you like to talk to people." he told her. "The only way to really learn is to take your own cases. If you get stuck you can always call on me."

She had always loved animals, so she started out treating horses and dogs, gradually expanding to treat friends and neighbors in her home ... people fed up with allopathic medicine ... and horse people. She thought of that period as her homeopathic internship with Henry Williams. "I treated the vet, then his wife, then his mother, his kids and finally all his friends," she remembered.

Then her MS began to get worse. As the twitching, tingling and numbness spread, she grew depressed and barely able to walk. So she came west to have her case taken by the homeopath she regarded as the best in America, Bill Gray. Under Bill's care, after heavy aggravations, Vicky soon began to feel better. "The weakness in my legs went away and so did my touchiness and obsession with diet. I was happier, more loving, and I no longer needed ten hours of sleep," she recalled happily. "I was euphoric. After all those bad years I was finally feeling well!"

"When I told Bill I wanted to practice homeopathy, he tried to talk me out of it. 'I wanted to see if I could discourage you,' he told me later. 'I had to test your commitment.' He's a very wise man. And he's the spirit of homeopathy in America right now, it seems to me."

Vicky enrolled in Hahnemann College because she knew she needed formal instruction. "I'd learned too much on my own and from books," she said. "It was wonderful to be able to meet and talk with the other doctors who were doing the same thing I was. We shared our problems and helped each other all we could. I learned a lot from my schoolmates." Vicky commuted to College from a part-time practice in Seattle where she shared quarters with a massage therapist and a chiropractor.

Like Matt she was hired by the Clinic right after she graduated.

Mark Rosen, DO (Doctor of Osteopathy), first heard of homeopathy in medical school when his instructors ridiculed all low strength medicines by sneering at them as "homeopathic." The earnest young Detroiter was studying to become an osteopathic physician at Michigan State University, "because it seemed an effective holistic means of facilitating the body's own healing capacities."

Mark defines osteopathy as manipulating the body to restore freedom of motion to damaged tissue, using a medical model of the body. "We see tissues disturbed that are disrupting flow," he explained, "and we work to re-establish fluid continuity in those tissues." But even as a student he was open to alternative methods of healing.

While in medical school he met a lay homeopathic practitioner who told him fascinating tales of miraculous cures and explained homeopathy's theory and origins. What had happened to Dr. Linda Johnston when Arnica cured her bruised knee ... and happened to Dr. Mark Vuksinich when he read Hanemann and Kent, now happened to Dr. Mark Rosen.

"I was drawn to homeopathy from the start, but afraid of it, too," he admitted. "The mass of information a homeopath had to learn overwhelmed me. But there was something about the philosophy that resonated with my sense of the laws of the universe. It inherently made sense to me to work with the whole person, to use small doses and to stimulate the body to heal itself."

"But it scared me, too," he said candidly, "so I hid out from homeopathy by taking a three year residency in psychiatry. By the time I was through I knew I wanted to learn more about holistic medicine, and I figured the Bay Area was the best place to go." So he moved west from Detroit to open an osteopathic practice in Palo Alto, California, in 1983. From the beginning he found his work satisfying.

"I love osteopathy because it's so immediate. I find it deeply gratifying to place my hands on my patients, to meld with them and guide them to a point of greater balance. It's an effective means of treatment and at times the changes are both fast and deep."

At the same time he cautiously investigated homeopathy. And he often met patients who had received great benefits from treatment at Hahnemann Clinic. The more he learned, the more the two approaches seemed harmonious and compatible. Before long he was spending all his spare time studying homeopathy. Although osteopathy had long ago "sold out," as he put it, to allopathy, it was still holistic and vitalistic in nature. Like homeopathy, it strives to stimulate the vital force.

"I see no conflict or contradiction between the two," said Mark. "The work I do osteopathically is not suppressive. I strive for a fuller expression of the vital force. But there are times when I'd also like to stimulate it medicinally. That's where homeopathy comes in. The difficulty is that, while I'm fairly accomplished as an osteopath and have a successful practice, I consider myself a mediocre homeopath. And I find it hard to charge for mediocre work. So I'm integrating homeopathy into my practice *very* slowly!"

There is ample precedent for combining the two arts. In the late nineteenth century, many osteopathic physicians were also homeopaths. And the English osteopath who introduced Mark to cranial manipulation was a homeopath who practiced both.

When Mark feels his osteopathic patient would benefit from homeopathic medicine, he explains what's involved and only prescribes after painstaking analysis. He was drawn originally to osteopathy because he liked the intimate contact with his patient. He finds the same kind of appeal in homeopathic casetaking. His psychiatric training also fits in nicely.

"At times a homeopath has to be a master psychologist," he pointed out. "He has to bring his patients to the point of tension, making them face their pathology at its height. At the same time he's observing them objectively. My psychiatric training gives me insights and deepens my relationship with the patient. I hear things

I might otherwise miss. I can interpret the way a patient talks and moves. Homeopathic and psychiatric interview techniques are very similar."

"When I used to try and study Boericke's or Kent's, work," he remembered, "every remedy picture looked the same. I'd say, 'This is ridiculous.' and put it down. Now I'm beginning to see the differences. It's still difficult but thanks to the professional instruction we received, now it's finally making sense."

Where Are They Now?

Linda Johnston, MD, has emerged as something of a media genius and spokeswoman for homeopathy. Lecturing, writing, traveling worldwide, making tapes and frequently appearing on radio and television, she is helping spread the good news of homeopathy.

"She's the best promoter homeopathy has had in years," says Bill Gray. "Her enormous success has proven that homeopaths don't have to starve, and that's invaluable when it comes to attracting good doctors to our field. But she's more than a promoter, she's a damn good homeopath. She was third in her class and she's very professional and humble. If she doesn't feel competent on a difficult case, she sends the patient to me, then does the followup. I'm delighted with her work."

Although she's still studying, Linda's Los Angeles practice is swamped, with a two year waiting list. The overflow and more difficult cases are directed to Hahnemann.

Dr. Matt Vuksinich, who put himself through Med School playing the mandolin, and Vicky Menear, the MD Bill Gray cured of MS, both began work on the Hahnemann Clinic staff as interns for six months. At the end of each day they went over each of their cases with either Bill or Roger. When their internships were over they received offices and patients, but continued to work closely with the Clinic's experienced physicians.

"It's the high point of my week when I get to sit down with Roger and discuss my cases," said Matt. "It's wonderful to be able to pick the brains of a great homeopath." Matt has remarried and he and his new wife each have two children, so he still has to work in an Emergency Room a couple of times a week to pay the bills, but he loves what he's doing. "When I came to work at the Clinic I got admitting privileges at two local hospitals, but in more than two years I haven't yet had to use them. We see very sick people, but homeopathy is so successful that hospitalization is rarely necessary."

Vicky works closely with Bill Gray, sharing his office. "I try to share myself with my patients," she told me. "It makes a big difference. I see their faces soften when I tell them of my struggles with MS. Homeopathy gets me into other people's worlds. That's the part I like the best. I love what I'm doing. I've never been happier in my life."

Dr. Mark Rosen, the osteopath integrating homeopathy into his Palo Alto, California, practice, has been highly successful combining cranial manipulation with homeopathic medicine.

7

Deanne's Constitutional

A New Remedy for Me ... The Dangers of Dental Drilling

Back home in the desert after a winter in Hawaii, Deanne complained that the climate change was aggravating her cough. Two weeks after returning we were in Hahnemann Clinic, Deanne for a constitutional, me for a followup. I was about to find out if my cure was working ... or I was merely deluded by Tuberculinum optimism.

After showing Deanne the Greek temple, I took her upstairs to Bill's office and introduced her. She sat down across from him, her face pink with excitement. She blushed a little as she told him about the sore throats and coughs that now came with every cold or change in climate. Her voice was husky from coughing. Her symptoms had become chronic five years before when a virus attacked her thyroid gland. Since then she had gone to various specialists who couldn't find anything wrong with her but gave her a lot of heavy drugs.

Bill asked her if she'd ever had headaches, intestinal troubles or stiff necks. She hadn't. When he shifted to food cravings she told him, "I really like chocolate—especially with caramel. With nuts it's even better!"

He smiled. "You're making me hungry!"

For forty minutes he questioned her closely about fears and phobias, sleeping habits, dreams, how she handled conflicts, arguments and criticism and things that worried her. He found out about a murder she had witnessed as well as the violent murder of her grandparents. The killings bothered her a long time and still made her apprehensive at night, especially when alone.

"Does it bother you if people are messy?" he asked her.

"No. I *do* like things neat, but mess doesn't bother me. Your desk is neat as far as I'm concerned."

"It looks neat to me, too," he quipped. "But wait 'til the end of the week."

After another ten minutes of questioning Bill re-read his notes, studied his Materia Medica and looked up, smiling.

"All right," he said briskly, "I can give you good news. You're very healthy. There're two possible remedies that should clear up what few problems you have. I can't confirm one of them so we'll go with the other. It's called Arsenicum. I think it fits overall. I don't see any need for a formal followup visit. You're going to get over this throat problem. I expect you'll just gradually get better."

She nodded. "We bought a home remedy kit it Hawaii. Can we still use it?"

"Good question. Since this remedy is chronic, you ought to be careful. Treating injuries is okay, but if you start treating flus you might get into the range of Arsenicum, and that could interfere. Better let me prescribe for you over the phone before you use your kit."

"Okay. What about menthol and herb teas? Some people say they'll antidote."

"I know. That's because menthol smells something like camphor. But the chemistry is entirely different. I've looked into it very carefully. Don't worry about teas or menthol."

"What about dental work? I've got an appointment next Tuesday. I know Robert can't have any drilling. What about me?"

"Theoretically it's the same, but for you it's not a big deal. If you antidote you'll recover very easily because your vital force is so strong. I rate it ten on a scale of ten. You've got a few minor problems, but not enough to grade you down to nine."

Now it was my turn. I had written out a timetable of the important events during our six months in Hawaii. Using it as an outline, I reminded him of the two courses of antibiotics I had taken and the return of my Tuberculinum symptoms after each.

Then came the mysterious aches and pains in my back that baffled the chiropractors. I paused, hoping for comment.

He nodded noncommitally. "What else?"

"Well ... I experienced a sort of ... personality change." I told him how I'd come to like cats, and had lost my craving for bacon.

"Really? That's perfect! Two keynotes changed. That's real confirmation. Your vital force kept on working, all right. That's great!"

"So what comes next?"

"You're doing very well. Normally, I wouldn't prescibe, but I think you're going to have a rough time in the coming pollen season. The Tuberculinum *could* help you, but I don't think it's going to be enough. So I'm going to give you Natrum muriaticum right now. It's a common remedy, but I think it will help. I'm giving you a low potency so if it doesn't work we still have time to go to something else. If it helps, we'll move up to a higher potency. Besides, we don't have to worry about Natrum mur antidoting the Tuberculinum."

That night Bill and Deanne and I went to dinner at a restaurant near the clinic. Bill told us Natrum mur had cured his migrane headaches and hay fever. He had been suffering so much that a grateful patient of his had flown him to Greece so George Vithoulkas could treat him. That was ten years ago. It had taken three years, but Bill's migraines and hay fever had never returned.

During dessert he confirmed that my muscular aches and pains in Hawaii had indeed been the return of old symptoms. "That's why the chiropractic adjustments you tried were useless," he explained. "Your vital force was methodically working it's way backward through old ailments."

He turned to Deanne, smiling. "Here's my chance to get some positive confirmation. Tell me about Robert and cats."

She corroborated my story.

"What about bacon?" he pursued.

"He still likes it," she reported. "But he doesn't ask for it anymore and sometimes he doesn't finish it. And only six months ago he was fighting our baby girl for every strip!"

Driving home to the desert with Deanne the next day, I began to wonder about the Natrum mur type. Deanne remembered it was included in the brief Materia Medica in the back of Vithoulkas' "blue book." Sure enough there were seven juicy pages on the remedy I shared with Bill ... written by him! But only half the symptoms applied to me.

A few days after returning, Deanne and I went to the dentist. Her teeth were perfect, but x-rays showed I had a sizeable cavity. "If you wait six months," warned dentist David Lund, "the nerve will be infected and you'll probabaly need a root canal instead of just a filling."

I told him I'd check with Bill. In the weeks that followed, no matter how I probed, I could find no evidence that the Natrum mur was working. Deanne, however, felt decidedly better since taking the Arsenicum. At first she'd been worse, suggesting a healing crisis, then her cough and sore throat had disappeared.

Four weeks later I called Bill to report the failure of the Natrum mur and ask if I could get my tooth filled before coming down for a new remedy. I was sure he'd be pleased with the timing, so I'd already made a dental appointment. But Bill surprised me by advising, "I'd strongly recommend against filling it. Drilling antidotes remedies very reliably. There's nothing worse than dental work."

"But what's to antidote?" I protested. "You said the Tuberculinum was finished.... And the Natrum mur doesn't seem to be working. It seems like we've got a perfect window...."

"Your window assumes an awful lot," he retorted. "What if I'm wrong about the Tuberculinum? And what if you're wrong about the Natrum mur? I won't know about that until I retake your case."

"But I can't ignore the decay! It isn't going to go away."

"Maybe it will. I've often seen it happen. The remedies and the body may very well take care of it. Dentists are demons for filling every little hole. Don't worry about something discovered on a routine examination from x-rays. That's my advice. Wait until the body tells you there's a problem. It'll warn you if work is really needed. You don't want to risk starting over just because your dentist wants to drill."

"What do you mean, 'start over'?"

"Well, typically, if you antidote, you lose one full layer. That wouldn't be so bad if it's the Natrum mur. But what if the Tubercu-inum's still working? You'd go back to craving bacon and hating cats. Your irritability would come back. And I'm afraid your rash might be worse than before."

I was thunderstruck. Risking a year's gains was unthinkable.

"It could be even worse than starting over," Bill went on. "When a remedy is antidoted, the symptom picture tends to be confused. It's often hard to get going again."

I groaned. "I had no idea of the risk," I confessed. "I'll cancel my appointment."

"That's what I'd do.... Tell me, do you still have the crotch rash?"

"Yup, it's still there."

"Hmmm. If the Natrum mur was working that should be gone by now. You may be right. You better come down and I'll retake your case."

After hanging up, I told Deanne the story. Bill had presented a shocking new concept: dentists were no better than allopaths! Everything they wanted to do might not be justified. Fortunately, I had time. I'd see Bill before going to the dentist, but anytime after that I could get the tooth filled if it started to hurt.

When I called Dr. Lund I asked for advice. He told me my decay was at the bottom of a food trap. "Food lodged between the teeth overnight provides a banquet for bacteria. Stop feeding the bacteria and you might double your time before you need a root canal ... or the onset of pain. But it means flossing after every meal, then rinsing with a flouride mouthwash."

I thanked him and went straight to the bathroom for a treat-ment. The race between decay and homeopathy had begun!

8

A Day in the Life
of Hahnemann Clinic

Cases of ... Chronic Indigestion ... AIDS ... Suicidal
Depression ... Alcohol & Drug Addiction ... Hay Fever
Allergy...Grief & Strain ... Severe Injury ...
Paraplegic Paralysis ... Catatonia

At 8:30 am on a fine May morning I stepped through the tall white
doors and climbed the stairs to Bill's office. After the briefest of
greetings he said, "Our first patient is hostile. She wouldn't let you
watch, so you may as well go talk to Roger."

An hour later he was back. "You didn't miss anything," he said
sourly. "All she did the whole time was complain about me and the
people at the desk."

When he paused, Roger asked his interpretation of a particular symptom picture. Bill willingly advised him, then asked questions of his own about a little-known remedy that Roger had seen
George use in Greece. They talked rapidly in homeopathic lingo,
exchanging technical information. It was all Greek to me. And it
was almost ten o'clock.

"Come on," Bill beckoned, heading for the door. "It's time for
our next patient." Back in his office, he hurriedly told me, "All I
know about Sandor is that he flew up today from Southern
California, and he claims to have seen me ten years ago. I don't
remember him."

Moments later a swarthy compact man with a middle European face and accent came in, bowed stiffly and sat down. With his tanned face and muscular body, Sandor reminded me of a Swiss ski instructor. He talked earnestly, leaning forward, his face serious, his body tense. He was fifty-one, he said, and a native of Poland. And he suffered terribly from digestive problems. "I have it all written out for you," he said, producing a packet of at least ten typed pages.

Bill smiled but made no motion to take the papers. "I'd rather you just answered questions," he coaxed.

"Then I will read," said Sandor firmly. Putting on his glasses, he haltingly began to read. "From the time I was born...." The style was formal and stiff and sounded like a textbook on his life. Bill listened impassively ... waiting. After several minutes the nervous Pole put down the papers and continued on his own. Bill seemed to have won....

Sandor had been born with poor digestion. Immediately after eating even the smallest amount of the blandest food he became so drowsy he was unable to work. To confirm his self diagnosis, he reported that his stools revealed no sign of food digestion. "If I eat carrots, out comes carrots. If I don't eat, I'm great. My health is fine. I'm unusually strong and active for my age. But as soon as I eat I lose all energy. I have to lie down and go to sleep. And the trouble persists for many hours. What can I do? This is destroying my whole life!"

Bill asked specific questions about the foods he ate, variations in his symptoms, what made them better or worse.

Sandor evaded most direct questions, preferring to relate what he regarded as important, frequently digressing, repeatedly assuring Bill that he had studied his health carefully and knew exactly what was wrong with him. It was a continuous contest of wills.

When Bill's inquiry drifted toward mental and emotional symptoms, Sandor became even more fidgety and evasive. Bill responded by inserting light quips between probes. Deft questioning revealed that the slippery Pole hated criticism of any kind, was uncomfortable with groups, disliked intimacy but not sex, avoided discussing his problems and often felt irritable. We learned that he had been to many kinds of doctors, including an array of homeopaths, worldwide. He had even been treated by George Vithoulkas in Athens. In addition to their prescriptions, he had self-prescribed after exhaustive study of his various Materia Medicas.

Sandor was looser now and readily admitted to feeling constantly cold, being a victim of insomnia, to being a perfectionist who lived a disordered life and had a fear of heights. "I worry a lot. And I like to be alone. Frankly, people get on my nerves. I have a lot of quick romances, but never a long relationship. I have a great and unusual sensitivity to color. Amber always soothes my nerves. I can count on it."

I wondered if the hour wasn't nearly up and caught Bill sneaking a look at a clock hidden from Sandor's view behind some books. "All right," he said expansively. "I've figured it out. I'm going to give you a combination remedy I think will help. But you have to stop taking everything else or it won't work. And you must take it religiously three times a day!" He leaned forward, dead serious.

Nodding eagerly, Sandor rapidly scribbled notes. I couldn't believe I'd heard Bill prescribe a combination remedy! It was contrary to everything he'd told me. "Combos are for quacks," he'd always insisted, "never for classical homeopaths!"

The moment Sandor was out the door, I started to protest, but Bill silenced me with a gesture. As he picked up the phone he muttered in my direction, "This is going to shock you, I'm afraid." Then he barked into the phone, "Michael! You're about to get a prescription for Calc sulphuricum!" he told the pharmacist down the hall. "Give him Sulphur 200 instead! Got that? Sulphur 200!" He hung up and leaned back in his chair, looking grim.

"I hate to be deceitful, but there's no other way. His case is all messed up. He's a 'doctor hopper.' There's been far too much prescribing. His only hope is to replace all this chaos with a systematic approach. The first thing he'll do is look up Calc sulphuricum in his Materia Medicas. He'll find some vague references that will probably satisfy him, so he'll take it. If he knew it was Sulphur he wouldn't give it a chance because he's already tried it and it didn't seem to work—probably because he didn't wait long enough or he antidoted it or mixed it with something else."

I had been momentarily stunned by the sudden turn of events, but his explanation made sense and his action seemed justified.

"I've got to gain his confidence before I can help him," Bill went on. "It's a tricky case. I don't know if I can cure him because I don't think he'll stick around long enough. Sulphur should help, but I think he'll eventualy need Lycopodium. He was a tough nut to crack, but that could fit either Lycopodium or Sulphur. He's theorized himself to death and that fits Sulphur better. And he's got enormous confidence in his judgement. I could bulldoze or confuse a Lycopodium. I couldn't do that with him. He'd leave if I got too hard."

He glanced at the hidden clock. It was eleven o'clock and time for the next patient. But before Bill could fetch her a buzzing on his desk told him there was an urgent phone call. It was a young gay man calling from Utah. He had just been diagnosed as having AIDS. He'd heard about Bill and hoped he could help him. In his businesslike way, Bill fired rapidfire questions to ascertain the state of his health and the extent of his symptoms. When he was satisfied, he stated his conditions.

"I won't treat AIDS on a one-shot basis. You'd have to move closer. I'd need to see you monthly for at least six months. You'd have to get off your anti-depressants and all other drugs ... even the codeine you take for diarrhea. What do you think? Does that sound possible?"

The young man hesitantly thought it might be.

"Good. You sound treatable to me—but not by phone. You need to understand that you're very sick. This is serious, but not out of hand—yet. Our approach here is very different from your regular doctor's. It's another realm, really. We don't try to kill the virus, we get the body to expel it. We treat the whole person. Your weakened immune system benefits from that. I think I might be able to help you. I've had some good results with AIDS, but every case is individual. A lot depends on how hard you'll try. I'll have the desk send you some literature. Think it over and let me know. Okay?"

The young man thanked him and hung up.

Bill shook his head. "He heard about me from a Salt Lake City boy I've been treating for AIDS. I got that one too late. He's only in his twenties but he'll be dead in another year. I treated his mother successfully for asthma, but he waited too long before coming. Many AIDS types live in an unreal world. They seem incapable of taking their disease seriously—until it's too late." He shook his head.

He'd had six AIDS patients, he told me, who had been following directions and gradually recovering, when one after another they'd all gone back on drugs and antidoted their remedies.

"Mostly they take antibiotics for venereal disease. They use a lot of penicillin. You wouldn't believe how much. But sometimes the problem's Amyl nitrate. They sniff it to enhance their orgasms and it antidotes their remedies. So does the coffee they can't seem to stop drinking. Their vital forces often aren't too strong, so they tend to antidote easily. They haven't the stability to deny themselves. The ones I get early enough—who follow directions—do okay. A few are free of symptoms and I've got four right now who are steadily getting better. The guy who just called could probably make it. It's early enough. It all depends on him." He shrugged.

He glanced at the clock and abruptly shifted gears. "This next lady tried to kill herself last week. Bella's highly psychotic. She'd been to see me just before she did it. I gave her Mercury, and apparently she took it. Then she OD'd on sleeping pills. They put her in the hospital and pumped out her stomach. . . . I'll go get her."

He returned with an anorexic looking woman in her forties dressed in baggy jeans, sneakers and a plaid flannel shirt. Bella walked like an invalid, without a vestige of spirit. She sat down resignedly, her hands limp in her lap. She seemed utterly passive and hopeless. Treating her kindly, Bill inquired about her health in a general way, gently urging her to respond, apparently measuring her mood before matter-of-factly asking why she'd tried to kill herself.

"It was in my mind even before I came to see you last time," she replied in a monotone. "I couldn't go home. I have no home anymore." She roused herself then to complain bitterly about the treatment she'd received in the hospital, speaking articulately in the jargon of one who's spent a lot of time with psychotherapists.

"They turned me into a zombie with their damn anti-depressants. I didn't want them, but I felt powerless to refuse. They ignored my acute depression, my deep pain. All they cared about was maintaining their damn hospital schedules and routine! The paramedics even dropped me on my tailbone. It's still sore."

Bill put gum in his mouth and began chewing vigorously. I'd never seen him do that before. Leaning forward over the desk, chin in hand, he asked casually, "Are you thinking of suicide again?"

She nodded. "But not with pills." She meaningfully ran her fingernails across her wrists. "I feel lost without friends. I feel like I'm not really here. My movements have turned slow. Part of me is numb. I don't feel real anymore. I'm disoriented. All I can eat is gentle foods, like tea and soup—and eggs. I eat eggs because the protein is non-fattening." Further questioning revealed that she feared getting fat! Bill probed her eating habits in detail, then asked about feelings of anger and cruelty.

Suddenly she exploded. "I have a deep rage that I'll never express!" Bella snarled. She clenched her small fists until they trembled. "Sometimes I just want to kill, kill, kill! It comes out over and over in my writing." She pounded one skinny fist on the desk. "I can't help it. It's the kids. They'll never forgive!"

Bill sat upright. "The kids? What kids?"

She hesitated, apparently embarrassed. "They're the part of me that feels, I guess. At times they take over, then I get mad. That's when I go out in the sun. The sun helps me relax. It makes me let go. The kids feel they have to get sick to get attention. When they get wild I have to call on 'control.'"

"Control?" Bill gently prodded.

'Control' is another side of me. He got us through childhood, back when it wasn't safe to go to sleep. Sleep means letting go, and that's scary. Sometimes I wake up with searing headaches." She suddenly grabbed her head. "Just mentioning it has brought one on!"

"What kind of headaches? And where?"

She pointed to her sinuses and eyes. "I get all kinds, sometimes even migraines." Out of the blue, she added, "The remedy

116

you gave me made me feel better. After I took it I had a feeling of lightness, a lifting sensation."

When Bill probed for details she changed the subject, telling him of her hypersensitivity to loud noises and bright light. She explained how sensitive her hair was to changes in her mood and stress levels. Her current mood, she said, was depression. Timidly she reached out her hand and Bill took it. "You're in a bad spot," he said gently. "But I think I can help you. I've got a remedy that speaks to a lot of your problems: inner conflicts, rage, desperation, separation. It should lift you out of your depression."

Tears flooded her eyes and ran down her cheeks.

"Don't be afraid to hope. Come back in two weeks and we'll see. By then you should be better—and better able to deal with your problems—one at a time. I'm giving you both a long-lasting high potency dose and a daily low potency dose. I want you to take it every day with your sleeping pills, but not more than one dose each day. That's important. Understand?" He leaned forward, intent.

Bella nodded submissively, reminding me of an obedient child about to dutifully take her medicine. But when she left there was a trace of spring in her step.

After closing the door, Bill told me he'd given her Anacardium orientale, made from a nut. When he read to me from Kent's Materia Medica about the remedy's symptom picture, I immediately understood his questions about cruelty and eating. Both involved Anacardium keynotes. Then the buzzer again directed him to pick up the phone.

It was a woman in Kansas he once had cured of hay fever. She was calling for her son, who was dependent on alcohol and drugs. Bill was blunt and concise.

"Tell him I'll help, but he has to quit drugs and come in for regular visits. And he has to call to make his own appointments. Don't do it for him. Homeopathy requires self-examination, honesty and desire. He has to participate if he wants to get well. I'll have the desk send you some material for him to read. But tell your son he has to make the decison and take the initiative. Otherwise it's a waste of everybody's time."

He hung up and shook his head. "It's a bad sign when a relative calls. It usually means the patient's not well motivated," he told me. "It's bad news that he's on alcohol and drugs, with a schizophrenic background to boot. We rigorously discourage dependency in patients. We want people who will take responsibility for their lives. They stand a much better chance of getting well."

It was now twelve thirty and Bill had a date for lunch, so we parted until his next appointment at 2 pm. I returned to the Clinic early to visit Peggy Chipkin, RN, FNP (Registered Nurse, Family Nurse Practitioner), to whom Bill had introduced me earlier. She too was a homeopath, but while he dealt mostly with long-term cures of chronic problems, she primarily prescribed acute remedies for immediate family aches and pains.

Her medical education, she told me, had begun with nursing school, where she got her RN. Pharmacology school came next. But she soon grew disenchanted. "It appalled me to read labels that listed ten side effects on every popular drug. That was just too many." She didn't care for hospital nursing either, so she was ready for something new. She met an acupuncturist who also practiced homeopathy, and he gave her Vithoulkas textbook, *The Science of Homeopathy*, to read. "It got me thinking about family homeopathic treatment."

Looking for homeopaths, she met Bill and he took her on as his apprentice. For the next several years she sat in with his patients, attended his classes and study groups, and read all she could. When Bill went to Greece she took over his easier cases while working and studying at Hering Clinic. When Bill returned, she joined him in practice, later completing work for her FNP. Now she's a full-fledged classical homeopath, specializing in the treatment of children for acute ailments.

Before 2 pm I was back in Bill's office, where he told me about Paula, his next patient. "She's got an undiagnosed neurological disorder. I've treated her for years—with very poor results." He shook his head. "Two years ago George took her case and gave her Natrum mur. That helped but a year ago she antidoted—with alcohol. She only took one drink." He shook his head.

"I thought alcohol didn't antidote. Is her vital force low?"

"No, she's a seven out of ten. It's rare, but it happens.... She called last week to say she was worse. I'm worried about her. I've *got* to find a way to help her!" He got up to go get her. Moments later I heard laughter in the hall and Bill ushered in an attractive woman of forty-four wearing a colorful sweater, skirt and blouse. Both of them were smiling at some joke they had shared. "Okay," Bill turned serious. "Tell me what's been happening. We've been doing this so long, you know all my questions."

She consulted a dog-eared notebook. "I'm afraid I've taken a big downturn," she said seriously. "I've had a gradual return of my chills, dry mouth, anxiety and inability to sleep. And I get twitching, on and off, all over my body. Sometimes they're like tics. Sometimes it's actual trembling. And I have trouble with my thermostat. One day I'm cold, the next day I'm hot. "The worst part," she continued, "is that I keep getting worse. My anxiety's rising. I feel so cut off. I keep losing a little more."

She held up one hand, then the other, to show him. I could see a faint trembling in both.

"It used to be entirely on my left side, then my right leg started tingling last summer. Now it's spread to the back of my right arm. My shakes don't go away like they used to. Why do I get worse every time I take a remedy?" Her voice was mildly plaintive, but not whining or accusing.

"Because so far we've failed," Bill said with a grimace. After questioning Paula about her tingling and shakes, he asked about her energy.

"I guess it's pretty good," she chuckled. "I just painted a three bedroom house all by myself. But I'm edgier all the time. I find myself snapping more at Janet (her daughter). And at times I find myself close to collapse at work. It's harder now to hide it when the shakes come on. I get anxious and confused. My anxiety soars. Sometimes I have to go lie down."

"Are you worried about your job? Is this interfering with your performance?"

"No. Luckily, I'm left alone—as long as I get my job done. So far I've been able to keep up. People don't seem to notice the rapid trembling in my hands because it's so faint. But I find my left leg

119

starts jiggling when I sit with my heel lifted." She demonstrated. Sure enough, her leg began to jiggle as soon as she lifted her left heel. Bill nodded grimly and she went on.

"These attacks—or downturns as I think of them—sometimes last for hours, sometimes days. I don't get any warning. Suddenly I've got the shakes. I haven't been able to make any association—except maybe with stress. I have more apathy now. I find it harder to function. I seem to sigh a lot. I feel I'm not getting enough air." She stopped to consult the notebook. "Oh, yes, my hair is dry and falling. I wake up at 4 am and can't get back to sleep. And sometimes I feel on the edge of hysteria."

She read another entry and giggled.

"What's that about?" Bill asked.

She hesitated. "Well . . . I went out with this man. He was quite a bit younger." She sounded embarrassed. "It was nothing romantic. But when he brought me home he gave me a goodnight kiss. I was so shocked I just stood there, on the edge of hysteria for a full ten minutes after he left. I didn't know whether to laugh or cry! It was very strange."

Bill nodded and opened his Materia Medica. He appeared to be studying three different remedy pictures. Finally he seemed to make a decision. "Here we go again," he said genially. "I haven't given you Phosphoric acid before, so let's try it. There's a reference to twitching muscles that sounds intriguing."

"By now it's probably the only thing I haven't tried," she tried to joke.

He smiled. "I still think your ultimate cure will come from Natrum muriaticum, but first we have to get you back on the track. It's a matter of timing. In a month, if the Phosphoric acid pulls you out of this, we'll try cranial osteopathy. I don't like the progression of your symptoms any better than you do. So the first thing to do is reverse the trend."

He gave her the prescription and got up. At the door he put a hand on her shoulder. "Hang in there," he said affectionately. They seemed more like old friends than doctor and patient. When she was gone Bill's smile turned to a frown. "I've *got* to find a way to help her!" he said with feeling. "No matter what I do, she keeps getting worse. I don't know how many hours I've spent thinking about her case. The eighty-five percent we cure are easy to forget. It's the fifteen percent failures that I see in my dreams!" He sadly shook his head.

It was now three o'clock. The next patient was new and from out of town. "It sounds like a routine acute case. Why don't you go talk to Michael?" I walked down the hall to Hahnemann Pharmacy, a commercial enterprise within but separate from the Clinic. In the window stood the proprietor, Michael Quinn. He was telling me that twenty basic homeopathic remedies accounted for fifty percent of all the prescriptions he filled, when suddenly Bill ran up and beckoned for me to come. "She's an allergy case," he told me. "Sounds interesting."

In his office he introduced me to Carol, an attractive blond woman of about thirty-five, dressed in a lavender sweater and matching skirt. Even the notebook on her lap was lavender. She wore glasses and appeared to be four or five months pregnant. Carol was suffering from acute hay fever, but she'd be moving back home to Montana in a month. She wondered if the change to high altitude would help. She spoke in a husky voice, complaining that her sore throat and drainage affected her speaking.

"Everyone hopes a move will cure their allergies," Bill observed. "It might give you two to four years relief, but then you become allergic to whatever's at the new location." After patiently listening to a brief account of Carol's common symptoms, Bill began sleuthing for her homeopathic picture. She answered him briefly and without emotion, as though taking an exam. She sat quietly but seemed to radiate tension. Her voice was getting hoarser and she began to twist a hankerchief in her lap, out of Bill's sight.

It soon came out that she'd been County Nutritionist and was a strict vegetarian. Bill appeared to grow more interested and questioned her closely while concealing that he'd been a nutritionist himself. Moving imperceptibly from the physical to the mental and emotional, Bill asked obliquely about family life with her husband and daughter. She replied appropriately but without much feeling. Bill brought out that she was somewhat disorganized, a bit forgetful and slightly sloppy. She said she needed twelve hours sleep every night when she was pregnant. I could see her feet twisting and turning beneath her chair.

Bill appeared perplexed. "When you lived in Montana, was your hay fever bad enough to take medicine?"

"I took Actifed." She brightened. "And once I took my baby to a homeopath for her allergies. The woman said the medicine would help me, too, but it didn't."

"What did she give you?" Carol couldn't remember.

Bill looked grim. "I can't do an acute treatment since you've already been allergic in Montana. We'll have to treat your chronic condition." His questioning now took a different line. Gradually it came out that though she professed to be vegetarian, she craved big juicy hamburgers.

"I think of them all the time," she confessed. "And sometimes I break down and buy one. I ought to be eating beans, but I'm sick of the smell of them cooking. I just can't eat them anymore—not since I've been pregnant."

She also admitted that she wasn't happy to be pregnant again. "I was in great shape before. I like exercise and I need it. Now I just can't work it in. I'm too busy with the kids." It turned out that her two-year-old was retarded and needed a great deal of care, and her husband wanted to live way out in the country while she preferred civilization. Carol's feet now seemed painfully contorted beneath the chair and she was mercilessly twisting the hankerchief in her lap.

Bill surprised me by telling her that taking homeopathic remedies meant giving up coffee. He was usually content to let Michael explain that. When she merely nodded, he prodded, "How many cups of coffee a day do you drink?" He smiled reassuringly. "Six or seven?"

She reluctantly nodded.

Bill sat back and changed the subject to nutrition. As they talked amiably, Carol stopped twisting her handkerchief. And her feet beneath the chair returned to a normal position. But her voice had gone dead and I thought she must be tired. Bill extracted her promise to return for another visit just before leaving for Montana. Then he gave her a prescription and she left.

The moment the door closed behind her he pounced. "I *knew* something was wrong from the start!" he said triumphantly. "There had to be some conflict she was hiding. She seemed to be expressive but her eyes were dead. I pegged her as Sepia from the location of her cold sores (left side) and the bleeding from her nose (right side), not to mention her slowness to warm. Those are all closed signs. But I almost missed it because she seemed to be expressive. She was expressing but not expressive. It's subtle, but there's a difference."

"What's Sepia like?"

"Carol's not so bad, but a full-blown Sepia woman's a cold-hearted bitch who lives in a half dead state. She only gets stimulation from kinky sex, anger and pain. She's totally apathetic the rest of the time." When I told him about the way she twisted her feet, he said, "She did that to induce energy. Sepia is *completely* apathetic. Dead inside. It takes something extreme to stimulate them. They have to induce pain in order to stay with the intensity of the interview. The pain takes the place of anger, perverse sex—or coffee."

I shook my head in wonder.

"These people need coffee to get through the day." Bill went on. "That's why I pressured her. If I was right about Sepia, she'd be a coffee drinker—no matter what diet she followed. When she admitted she drank it, that was the final confirmation. Sepia will work," he said with conviction.

He looked at the clock. It was past four-thirty. The four o'clock patient, another new one, had been waiting half an hour. "We better get going," he said briskly, getting up to fetch her.

Moments later he led Nan into the office. Small, lean and wiry, she had a serious pleasant face and hastily combed red hair. She wore old but clean cotton pants, a baggy sweatshirt and flipflops on her feet. She seemed to move uncertainly and sat down rather gingerly. Bill soon learned that she was forty-three, lived in the college town of Davis and had been urged to come see Bill by close friends he had helped.

"So what seems to be bothering you?" he asked.

She held up a surprisingly big, strong-looking hand and slowly bent her left forefinger. "It's painfully swollen, just like my left toe. When I get up in the morning, I ache in all my joints. I'm so stiff I can hardly move. It takes me an hour of painful manipulation to get loosened up enough to go to work." Her strained manner of speaking seemed to echo the struggle she was describing. And I've got severe hay fever and tender spots in my back and neck." She turned her body and reached around to point out the exact locations.

Bill nodded, waiting, and she went on.

"I'm macrobiotic, and that used to hold down the symptoms—if I was really strict. But after seven or eight beers at a party I'm a mess the next morning, with raging hay fever and crippling aches and pains. I realize now that diet will never cure me. Besides, I just can't stay on it."

Bill nodded. "It's a tough diet. When did this start?"

"It all began seven or eight years ago ... after my hysterectomy. I had a boyfriend at the time who really tore me up emotionally. About that time I quit smoking, and that was hard on me, too. I also had an operation for a stomach hernia." She shook her head sadly and sighed.

"Tell me about the boyfriend. What was the problem?"

She looked a little embarrassed. "I fell in love with my drinking buddy," she said simply. "I guess I needed him in some weird way, so it was hard to break up. I hated him and loved him. He treated me terribly, but I couldn't seem to leave him." She sighed. She had already been married and divorced twice and had three children. But this was the first man she had lived with "in sin," and her parents had made her feel very guilty about it. In fact they disowned her and refused to communicate.

"I finally got rid of him, but after that I never seemed to be able to pull my life together. I still feel guilty and lonesome, but I'm scared now of men. I blame myself for what happened to my daughter. She was ... molested by her older brother."

"What exactly happened?"

All this time she had been sitting motionless and erect, her hands limp in her lap, her feet flat on the floor. "My fourteen year old son tried to force himself sexually into my five year old girl," she said in a strangled voice. Now that she'd revealed her secret she seemed to relax. She sat back in the chair and let her feet slide forward. "After that I sheltered my daughter fiercely. Now I'm trying to undo that excess by pushing her to join groups and spend time with her friends."

Bill nodded and asked about her current life. She owned a cleaning service, she said, of which she was the sole employee. With the college semester ending, she was now under tremendous pressure to clean dozens of student apartments. The fatigue and her ailments made her feel so spacey and shaky that sometimes she had to sit down to keep from fainting. Her anxiety about her life and her various ailments made her stutter and gave her cramps. She felt on the edge of a nervous breakdown.

"Do you find it hard to relax?"

"*Very!* I have to be busy ... or I worry too much."

Bill asked if she ever took a real vacation, like two weeks on the beach at Hawaii. When she said she never had, he asked why? Couldn't she afford it?

Nan admitted that she could. "I guess I'm a workaholic. I wish I *could* relax." She sounded a little embarrassed.

"With all this business, why don't you hire helpers?"

"I tried that once. It was a disaster. I can't find anyone I can depend on to work to my standards, so I have to do everything myself." She sighed.

"How are your relationships nowadays?"

"Well, I don't go out much. I'm nervous about men and I haven't got much time. But after not speaking to me for thirteen years, my father is friendly again. That just started three weeks ago and I'm happy about it. And I've resolved my problems with my mom.... But I worry about my health. I gain water weight every time I go off the diet. I know there must be *some*thing I can do to get well ... I'd do *any*thing!" She looked at him imploringly.

"I believe we can help you. Do you have constipation?"

"Yes! Since birth! How did you know?" Her eyes were wide.

"What about menstrual cramps?"

"That's always been a problem, too! I often have two periods a month." She sighed. "After my boyfriend and I broke up, I hemorrhaged so heavily I had to go to the hospital."

Bill asked more about her childhood and learned she'd had to work very hard in school just to get C's. Her poor eyesight had been blamed. It wasn't discovered until she was a teenager. By then she was way behind with her schoolwork.

"Do you cry easily?"

"Very! I've got a lump in my throat right now!"

"And you sigh a lot?"

"Yes!" She looked at him in wonder.

"Okay," Bill turned businesslike. "I'm going to give you two remedies: one for emotional relief and your fatigue. Then a constituional remedy for your workaholic and worrying tendencies."

"I'm *ready!*"

He wrote out the prescriptions and told her to avoid hot mineral baths, which sometimes antidoted what he was prescribing. Though she was grateful and pleased, she got out of her chair stiffly and walked gingerly to the door.

As soon as she was gone Bill eagerly began his post-mortem, rubbing his hands together briskly. "That was a good case. I wish I had it on video for my classes. After thirty seconds in the waiting room I knew her vital force was low.

I only give her a three. She's a slow plodding person who can't take much stress. You heard what a hard time she had in school. She can work but she can't relax or delegate authority. When she got in a traumatic relationship eight years ago, all hell broke loose and her body started falling apart. The essence of her case now is grief, and that's an acute condition, so I'm giving her Ignatia. Then we'll go to Calcarea for her fundamental problems, her workaholic nature."

"I could feel you zeroing in on her picture," I chortled. "She thought you were some kind of magician."

"Once I got a sense of her, I could start asking questions to confirm or deny certain remedies. I knew she was Ignatia after only twenty minutes. Her cramping, sighing and grief all confirmed it, but her childhood constipation is what nailed it down for me. This is homeopathy at it's scientific best. These remedies, in time, are going to change her life." Even at the end of a grueling day, his enthusiasm for homeopathy was undiminished. And he clearly enjoyed doing post-mortems before a live audience. He glanced at the clock. It was nearly six.

With the last patient gone, it was time to answer the accumulated phone calls. Bill studied the call slips the office had brought him. Then he clipped them to the appropriate files for quick reference and set to work returning phone calls. First came a worried mother, reporting on her son. After listening for a minute, Bill said, "Don't let the symptoms upset you. In homeopathy symptoms are good, not bad. Sounds to me like he's better." His voice was kind. "I want you to stop giving him the remedy. If he starts to decline, let me know."

Next was a fifty-two year old man who had been in a wheelchair since childhood. Bill had been treating him for years and they were friends. He flew all over the world directing a rehabilitation program for the disabled. Yesterday, he told Bill, flight attendants had dropped him at the Philadelphia airport, causing severe bruising and pain.

Bill put him on hold and called to see if Michael had left. When the pharmacist answered, Bill asked him to please stay long enough to make up a couple of prescriptions. Then he told the patient, "Get someone to come down here right away and pick up your medicine. It'll be taped to the front door within fifteen minutes. It's late and Michael's anxious to go home. Take the Arnica right away for the shock and pain, then Rhus tox four hours later for the torn ligaments. And take it easy."

Bill grabbed a fresh file and dialed another number. The patient was obviously anxious and did most of the talking. It was twenty minutes before Bill hung up, shaking his head. "Here's a thirty-nine year old man, as healthy as you or me two weeks ago. Then he fell fifteen feet off a ladder while he was pruning a tree. It wiped out his spine. Now he's paraplegic—paralyzed from the waist down. They've got him in a rehabilitation center. That's the bad news."

I shuddered. "There's good news?"

He smiled. "I gave him Rhus tox as the first step. He says his bladder function has returned and they've already taken away his catheter and bag. And now he's got a sense of where his left foot is. That's an early sign that sensation's coming back and his spine is healing. Sounds like he's on the way to recovery. He says his rapid progress has blown the staff away. At first, they told him it was hopeless. Now they're sending him home! He chuckled.

I felt relieved. "Was it a tough diagnosis?"

"No, easy. This isn't disease. It's massive trauma, sure, but it's still an acute condition. This is just the first remedy. I'll be giving him others. It'll be a few weeks before we see how well the spinal nerves regenerate after the swelling goes down. But the early signs are good."

The next call was hard to decipher. Bill mostly listened, only contributing a few cryptic phrases. But as soon as he hung up he began to swear. "Damn it all to hell! Another freak antidoting. I can't believe it!" I had never seen him so upset.

After a minute he cooled down and told me the story. Liz had been catatonic, contorted and immobile, unable to eat or talk, from the age of thirteen. Bill had taken her case three years back, when she was twenty-one. In less than a year, he had Liz living a normal life, going on hikes, holding a job and supporting herself. She even had a boyfriend.

"Now her father tells me she got a mild shock off the garbage disposal two days ago and immediately began to regress. Fast! She's completely catatonic again. She antidoted a couple of layers, just like that." He snapped his fingers. "She's back where she started, her head pulled over to one side, with one arm up, the wrist bent." He demonstrated the grotesque position. "Actually she's *worse* than before! She's regressed from point zero! The poor kid. She can't talk, of course, but just imagine what she's thinking!"

"What can you do?" I half whispered, shocked.

"I've ordered Ignatia, her first remedy, in three dosages: one thousand, ten thousand and fifty thousand potencies, to be given to her one day apart. Her dad's coming to get them. They'll bring her back in a hurry."

"Bring her back? From worse than point zero?" It didn't seem possible.

"Today is Monday." he said. "I promise you she'll be completely normal by Thursday. Call me Thursday night and I'll tell you how she is." There wasn't a hint of doubt in his tone. I had to believe him.

He tilted back in his chair, weary but smiling. "'The thrill of victory, the agony of defeat,'" he quoted. "It's all in the day of a homeopath." He sighed and got up to put on his coat. It was 7:15 and the Clinic was empty. It was time to lock up and go to dinner.

Case by Case Follow-Ups

A year has passed and it's time to take a look at the lives of the patients Bill saw or talked to on that memorable day in May at the Clinic.

Sandor, the doctor-hopping Pole who had written his own interview, did well on the Sulphur that Bill tricked him into taking.

The gay AIDS victim who phoned from Utah, came to the Clinic for treatment. He responded well to his remedy and was greatly improved after only three weeks. Then he mysteriously went downhill. He finally admitted he'd never stopped taking his Codeine and prescription antidepressants. They effectively anitdoted his homeopathic remedy, leaving him extremely ill. Despite three units of blood, his condition appears terminal. Rather than start over, he went home to his mother in Utah.

Bella, the anorexic psychotic who had attempted suicide just the week before, made a dramatic turnaround in just two weeks under Bill's guidance. With the help of Anacardium orientale, she miraculously turned from suicidal desperation to volunteer work in several psychiatric clinics. Although she continued to compulsively binge on food and take sleeping pills every night, her "searing" headaches disappeared and most of the time she felt cheerful. "She's a changed person," said Bill, "and she'll keep getting better."

Paula, the courageous lady with the undiagnosed neurological disorder that made her hands and feet tremble, was helped by the Phosphoric acid Bill gave her and by the subsequent Cranial osteopathy. Her energy and emotional outlook improved but the tremors remained. George again took her case and prescribed Calcarea, but she put off taking it because she needed a lot of dental work. Three months in the dental chair disrupted the case and undid all her gains.

Bill waited several months to let her system settle before he started over, re-taking her confused case in the most minute detail. This time he used a computer programmmed with *MacRepertory*, the software developed by the Clinic's David Warkentin, another Hahnemann homeopath who studied with Vithoulkas in Greece.

"I spent at least half an hour just ranking her symptoms in order of importance before I started," Bill explained. "That's the key to using the computer successfully. That's why the computer's no substitute for skill and experience. It's only as good as the data you put in."

"What did the computer tell you?"

"Something very strange. I was doing what's called an Elimination *Repertorization*. Symptom by symptom I asked the computer for remedy pictures that were present in all her symptoms. Usually you can only go three or four symptoms deep before you get an answer—or a dead end. But with Paula's picture I was able to go eight! That's very rare. Only one remedy emerged, and it came out very strongly. It was Natrum muriaticum—again."

"George's original remedy?"

"Right. It was working nicely when she antidoted it with alcohol. I gave it again, in higher and higher potencies, but it never worked. I went up to 50M, with no results. I was bewildered. That's why I sent her back to George. He couldn't understand it, because he came up with Natrum mur, too. Calcarea was only his second choice."

"I don't get it."

"My conclusion, now, is that she was Natrum mur all along . . . and those high potency remedies I gave her just weren't any good! Since Michael's potent remedies had just become available, I was able to start over with a proven dose of Natrum mur 200. It worked. Her energy and emotional state are much improved. The tremor is about the same but it doesn't concern her now because she feels so good.

"The computer work was crucial. I had given up on Natrum mur, but the computer brought it back so strongly that I couldn't ignore it. So, now we've got an unbeatable combination—skilled homeopaths, the latest computer technology and Michael's dyna- mite remedies."

"Weren't you anti-computer just last year?"

"That's true. I'm still basically anti-data. It can easily be a trap. People get so carried away with data that they forget they have to think, too. They have to make correct deductions and plug them in correctly, or the computer's useless ... or worse. I use it mostly to pick out rare remedies I might not otherwise think of. Essentially the computer thumbs through the book *for* me, so I can check out the possibilities faster. With a given amount of time and energy, I can try more combinations. Just the other day I prescribed a rare remedy that I don't really know because it popped up on the com- puter. Otherwise I wouldn't have considered it."

The next patient was Carol, the County nutritionist on her way to Montana. Since her problem was local allergies, there wasn't much reason for her to return, and she didn't.

The last patient that day was Nan, the wiry driven cleaning woman with hay fever and stiff joints. She was *much* better after the Ignatia, but still overworked and fatigued. Calcarea cleared those problems completely. She still works hard but now she dele- gates responsibility to employees. For the first time in her life she can permit herself to rest and take vacations. Feeling balanced and happy, she's seriously thinking of marriage!

Next came the day's accumulation of phone calls. Some were urgent and desperate, some patients were just checking in. The wheelchair-bound man who been dropped by flight attendants got great and immediate relief from the Arnica and Rhus tox Bill pre- scribed over the phone. The man paralyzed from the waist down just two weeks before when he fell off a ladder enjoyed swift recov- ery of feeling in his legs with the help of the Rhus tox Bill gave him.

Then came the phone call that chilled me! After eight years as a catatonic, contorted and unable to eat or talk, Liz had returned to a normal life after only a year of Bill's treatment. Then a mild electric shock caused a freak antidoting. In a matter of hours Liz once more became catatonic, with contortion and involuntary spasms! After re-prescribing Ignatia, her first remedy, and arranging for delivery, Bill assured me Liz would be normal within three days. And she was. The spasms stopped within minutes of taking the Ignatia. Three days later, the catatonia was gone! Liz's now so active and busy with friends that her parents complain they never see her!

9

A Radical Approach

The first Monday in June I was back in Bill's office. Before he
could get started I asked, "What made you give me Natrum mur?"

"That was kind of an intuitive prescription," he said vaguely.
"We needed a new remedy to get a jump on the pollen season ...
so I took a stab. I can't explain it beyond that."

"What about my tooth.... Since the Natrum mur didn't work,
can I get it filled now?" I had been faithfully brushing, flossing and
disinfecting after every meal to hold infection at bay, but I didn't
want to push my luck.

He shook his head. "I wouldn't. There's too strong a chance
the Tuberculinum is still working. Maybe you'll be lucky and the
tooth won't need filling."

I grimly nodded.

"Now then ... I've got an idea that's a little bit radical. I want
to give you what we call an isopathic remedy ... to give you sage
itself ... homeopathically prepared. It's more than coincidence that
sage helps consumptives, people who get tuberculosis."

"What about rabbit brush? My hay fever starts when the rabbit brush blooms."

"Okay, we can try to get some rabbit brush and mix the two together. Maybe an allergist in your area could supply it. We'd only need a tiny amount, less than one cc. If you can get it, we'll make a real high potency dose, a CM, and give it to you before the season starts."

"What's a CM?"

"It's a one hundred to one dilution ... repeated a hundred thousand times. Oh, oh! It usually takes six months to make. We'll have to ask Michael about that."

"Is the isopathic long lasting?"

"You'd probably take it every season—well beforehand. Then you'd probably go through the season without reacting. It would *not* interfere with your case. It's rare that an isopathic treatment fits into classical homeopathy. But this one does. It could even cure you permanently ... because the sage fits. You might not have to take it every year. Let's go talk to Michael."

In the pharmacy, Michael told us he was about to take delivery on a Skinner Machine that would make dilutions every two seconds —continuously, day and night. "I'll be able to make you a CM in a week," he said proudly.

In Reno I found an allergist who ordered both rabbit brush and sage antigens from a pharmaceutical supplier. I passed this news to Michael who said if all went well he'd have my CM isopathic remedy in the mail within three weeks.

It was now mid June and the desert was heating up. As soon as school was out we left the house on the river and moved up to the cabin for the summer. A week later Deanne and I were at neighboring Berkeley Camp, where our young friend Danny and I often played basketball. Danny's head was hanging. "I keep getting these wierd cramps in my gut," he complained. "I feel like I'm gonna puke, but I can't. I never know when it's gonna hit."

"Sounds like a case for Dr. Deanne," I said, turning to my wife. She'd never treated anyone outside the family, but she said she'd try and she asked him a few questions. Before leaving we invited Danny to come to the cabin for lunch the next day. Afterward Deanne would "take his case." When lunch was over Deanne was ready with her clipboard, kit and two home treatment books. She had done some reading and already had a preliminary diagnosis.

In recent months she had become quite adept at curing our ills with the tiny arsenal of homeopathic remedies we had brought back from Hawaii ... and augmented at Michael's pharmacy. We never thought any more of using aspirin, iodine or Vaseline. Now it was Hypericum, Arnica and Calendula. Using the Outline for Casetaking in Cummings/Ullman as a model, Deanne phrased her questions to fit Danny's complaints. She sought first to classify his abdominal pain. He said it felt "knotted" and "fairly sharp." It came at random but never at night. Weather and temperature seemed to have no effect. Changing position gave no relief, but light pressure on his stomach made it feel better. So did drinking cold water. And when Deanne asked him if he'd been unusually thirsty he almost shouted, "Yes!"

Just before an attack he suddenly felt hungry. "It's the strangest thing," he said. "It might be only an hour after breakfast, but suddenly I'm hungry as hell. Then the pain hits. My stomach knots up and I'm sure I'll have to puke. But nothing comes up."

His body would get warm just before an attack, and when it struck he'd feel "spacey." He wobbled his head and rolled his eyes to illustrate. He'd always been bothered by bright light and even slight noises. Deanne asked about constipation, trouble urinating and diarrhea in a clinical manner worthy of any MD. Danny denied all three.

When Deanne smoothly shifted from the physical to the emotional, Danny admitted he felt pressured and driven on the job. Being with people made him anxious, and he confessed that he kept his irritation and anxiety well hidden behind an easygoing exterior. With some hesitation he acknowledged that he hated to be questioned, and admitted a craving for fatty foods, alcohol and coffee—all of which he'd consumed on the previous weekend.

Dr. Deanne was hot on the trail. The way she rephrased a question and came back to key symptoms reminded me of Bill. I saw her put down one book and open the other to get a second opinion. "Okay," she said at last. "I think I've got it. One remedy fits better than all the rest. It's Nux vomica. 'Wants to vomit and can't' seems to me to be the key. In fact that's what the name means in Latin."

"What is it?" asked Danny.

"The seed of the poison nut tree."

"You want to give me poison nuts?" His eyes widened.

"It's incredibly dilute," she assured him. "It can't hurt you at all. But it ought to fix you up."

"Okay," he shrugged. "Sock it to me."

Deanne opened her kit, took out a tiny vial and neatly dropped four pellets under his tongue. Then she gave him a dozen more in a Ziplock bag and made him promise not to drink any coffee. He was instructed to take four pellets before bed, four more upon rising and the last four after lunch tomorrow. All told, case-taking, prescription and treatment had taken half an hour.

After Danny left I congratulated Deanne on her professionalism and asked exactly how she'd diagnosed.

"Well, I looked up 'Stomach and Bowel Problems' in one book and 'Digestive Problems' in the other ... and quickly read through them. Then I pinned down Danny's symptoms by asking questions from the checklist, and writing down the answers. The answers best matched Nux vomica. So that's what I gave him. Anyone could do it. It was easy."

The next morning, Deanne began to wonder about her patient, so we went to see him. Danny was beaming. "I feel *much* better," he told us. He'd had some queasiness walking home from the cabin and he still felt a little dull, but he hadn't had another attack. He had faithfully taken the medicine as directed and dutifully denied himself coffee. Deanne was elated. Three days later when we stopped by the camp, Danny bounded onto the basketball court completely recovered. "Dr. Deanne is wonderful!" he exulted. "She's my doctor forever."

Her success with Danny not only demonstrates the effectiveness of homeopathy, it shows how easily it can safely be used by untrained but motivated individuals to treat common acute problems. That's why there are so many lay prescribers in America, in addition to highly trained homeopathic physicians.

Unfortunately, anyone who ever attended a weekend seminar

can call him or herself a homeopath, and there is a sizeable group of what Bill calls "homeopathic quacks," people who prescribe high potency chronic remedies without the necessary training. These bunglers don't put people in the hospital the way allopaths do, but they create problems for experienced doctors like Bill, Roger and Peggy, who have to undo the mischief.

One morning on the cabin's back porch, sitting in the sun and feeding the squirrels, I asked Deanne about her changes in the two and a half months since Bill gave her Arsenicum. She still occasionally had some drainage down the back of her throat, but she remembered that it used to be continuous. "I don't seem to feel the cold quite as much, either" she said thoughtfully. "A swim in the lake used to chill me for hours. Now I warm up quicker."

"How about mentally and emotionally?"

"Well, I seem to feel better about myself. I'm more interested in doing projects, and I don't get so involved in other people's problems." She blushed a little. "And . . . my crazy-silly moods s 'em to come more often. I hope you don't mind,"

"I like them. You seem happy."

She nodded, smiling. "So do you."

"I am. Coming back here after a year, it's easier to see certain changes."

"Like what?"

"Well, for years it bugged me when motorboats went speeding past our dock. Now I can't be bothered to complain. And I've grown less competitive, too. I don't get as intense when I'm playing ping pong or bridge. Winning and keeping score aren't so important any more."

"What about the physical?" Now she was taking *my* case.

"There's been a big boost in my energy. I'm bounding up peaks that last summer seemed too tough to climb. And I'm able to come from behind to beat Danny at basketball. Last year I couldn't do that . . . and last year it mattered more. . . . And I've never felt more creative. I'm eager to get back to serious painting. . . . And putting up Gellie's tent this year seemed a snap. It used to drive me crazy."

"You *do* seem more flexible," she admitted. "Let's go canoe-

137

ing." Paddling along the lakeshore, I told her I couldn't help wondering what was happening to the tooth that Dr. Lund said was decaying . . . and Bill felt was okay. I religiously brushed and flossed four times every day and so far, I'd had no discomfort.

When the isopathic remedy was a week overdue, I called Michael. The Skinner machine still hadn't arrived, but was promised for later that week. I'd have my remedy in a week, he assured me. The week passed, then another. Deanne and I made a quick trip to Walker for supplies. Summer was far advanced and the deadly yellow blossoms of the rabbit brush were almost open. The sight made me sweat. It was vital, Bill, had said, to take the isopathic *before* exposure to the pollen. Another week and the dust would be blowing in the wind! I was thankful to escape back to Echo without symptoms. Clearly, I couldn't go back again.

On a mid-August descent to nearby Lake Tahoe, I was shocked to find rabbit brush blooming along the shoulder of the road less than two miles from the cabin! Hopefully, I'd be protected from its pollen by the prevailing west wind. In September, Deanne and Gellie drove home to start school. I was exiled again from my family, without a car. It would be more than two months before we left for Hawaii in early November. My future seemed to hang on the arrival—and efficacy —of the isopathic remedy.

The next day I began to experience sudden bouts of sneezing, accompanied by itching eyes. A rare east wind was blowing straight from that roadside rabbit brush two miles away! Now that my remedy was due momentarily, the damn pollen seemed to have won the race!

When the CM remedy was two weeks overdue I called Michael. "Your remedy went out today by UPS," he told me. "But I'm afraid it's not a CM. We had to make it on the old succussion machine and we only got 3,449 dilutions before the machine broke down."

At least something was on the way. "How soon before I can go down and test it out?"

"Just wait overnight. By then you'll have the full effect. It's rabbit brush and sage mixed fifty-fifty. Bill said to take five pellets and save the rest. I'm sorry it's not CM and sorry about the wait.

But remember, anything above a thousand dilutions is really a very high dosage."

On Friday the remedy arrived and I took it. On Saturday night after dinner we drove home to Walker, arriving near midnight. Moonlight revealed rabbit brush blooming all around the house. The sage was not yet in blossom. Last year, I remembered, my hay fever symptoms had erupted after only eighteen hours. Six hours later I was desperate to escape, ready to kill anything that stood in my way.

This year, after two full days hiding out in the house, I was still symptom free. Cautiously elated, I went for a stroll by the river with Deanne. At the last minute I grabbed my fly rod. For two hours we wandered downstream, enjoying the fall afternoon. I had first fallen in love with this country in the fall, and I had built a house on the river so I could fish for trout. By the time we returned I had six plump rainbows, and I hadn't sneezed once!!

After four nights without symptoms, I called Bill to report. He was delighted with my news. "It sounds like it's working. Of course it may not hold. This isn't a true curative remedy. It's actually suppressive ... it's just to get you past the season. Your vital force at some point will probably get strong enough to overcome and expel it. The important thing is not to take another dose until you have a real relapse. Give yourself several hours of heavy symptoms first."

As the days passed my hay fever gradually got worse. Soon I no longer felt like going fishing. During a lull in the storm we went back to Echo. Within three hours of our arrival, my symptoms disappeared. Since hopefully I wouldn't have to live in exile this autumn, we began to close the cabin for the winter.

Back home in the desert my symptoms all returned. My eyes itched most of the time, my nose was running and I was sneezing. I wasn't as bad as last year and I did get brief periods of relief, but I felt like I was losing it, so I took a second dose of the 3449. Within two hours there was a magical change. My nose cleared and my eyes stopped itching and streaming. Amazing!

But my euphoria was short lived. Six months had passed since dentist David Lund had said I'd probably need a root canal. Fresh x-rays seemed to prove him correct. "It's three to one that if we went in right now we'd find the nerve infected," he reported. "If you wait until the tooth starts to hurt the root canal may be painful. If you wait even longer we'd have to pull the tooth."

I reminded him of the danger of drilling to my remedy. He nodded. "You might ask your doctor about using a slow speed drill. It feels like a jackhammer and takes three times as long, but it runs at only thirty to forty rpms, instead of 25,000. The speed might make a difference." When I called Bill to report I expected a protest. I wasn't disappointed. "I'll bet that's exaggerated!" he said hotly. "I'd get another opinion. Most dentists are too eager to drill. They don't realize the harm they can do!"

When I told him about Dave's low speed drill suggestion, his tone changed. "Hmmm. That might work. High and low vibration frequencies seem to be safe. I've got a dentist using a 50,000 rpm drill that hasn't antidoted yet. And we know that low speed grinders used for cleaning teeth are safe. Go ahead and try it. Actually it's a good time since we're only suppressing right now. You might very well get away with it. Some people—a small per-cent—aren't antidoted by *any* amount of drilling."

"Okay ... Deanne's been bothered by the pollen, too. Can she take the 3449?"

"I wouldn't if I were her. Taking an isopathic *can* create the problem it's trying to treat. When I first started practicing in Sebas-topol I got famous in a hurry for stopping hay fever. I made high potency isopathic remedies from the local pollens and gave them to everybody. It stopped symptoms, all right, but in the long run it didn't cure anybody. Some people even got worse, moving from hay fever into asthma."

I sighed. "I was hoping there was no down side. I guess that's too much to expect."

"In your case there probably won't be, because your vital force is so strong. The people who got worse had weak vital forces. You've got the almost unique combination of a strong vital force and a specific identifiable disabling problem. It's a rare situation, and it invites this approach."

At Toiyabe Indian Clinic a few days later, I told Dave to go ahead with the low speed drill. As soon as he was done I anxiously asked myself how I felt about bacon and cats. Happily my feelings hadn't changed. The Tuberculinum had apparently survived! Dave also had good news. "I can't see any evidence that decay has reached the nerve. We're in luck, or maybe your homeopathy helped."

"So no root canal?"

"Not now, at least. If the nerve can fight off any bacteria that may have reached it ... and recover from today's trauma, it should survive."

That night my hay fever came roaring back. By the time I went to bed I was wheezing with asthma. The drilling had obviously antidoted the 3449, so I took another dose. In the morning I was fine, but the effects didn't last. Clearly the remedy was losing its effectiveness. Fortunately, Michael had made me a 10M potency, which had arrived the day before. And there were only five more nights before I could escape across the mountains to Berkeley. Soon after that we'd be moving to Hawaii.

Before leaving for Berkeley I took the last eight pellets of 3449. They had no discernable effect. The timing had been perfect! Efficacy and supply had ended simultaneously. Eight doses had gotten me through exactly five weeks. I opened the treasured vial of 10M and took four pellets. Within an hour I felt solid relief. By time to leave for Berkeley, I was nearly back to normal.

Driving across the Sierra by myself, my mind in neutral, the uniform pine forests that lined the road seemed monotonous. Then I realized the implications of that judgement. Pines were no longer holy! My taste in trees had apparently changed. Another Tuberculinum keynote was gone.

In Berkeley I planned to see Bill and join homeopaths from all over the world who were gathering to watch George Vithoulkas at work. I had a date with Bill for the opening session, when the Greek master would attempt to solve a case that had baffled Hahnemann's best prescribers. George was reputed to be a showman and a genius, so it promised to be a memorable event.

10

The Master Solves a Case

**George Vithoulkas on Stage Unearths Early Emotional
Trauma to Discover the Curative Remedy in A Difficult Case**

There were sixty of us seated at five rows of tables in the little conference room in Berkeley. The young lady to my left had come from Switzerland to watch George Vithoulkas work in hopes of better providing for her patients. Beside her, a keen-eyed man in a tan windbreaker sat idly tapping his foot, waiting for the program to begin.

To my right sat Bill Gray, his dog-eared *Repertory* propped on a folding stand, his waterstained Materia Medica with the broken binding open in front of it, ready. The audience consisted mainly of homeopaths and students at Hahnemann College of Homeopathic Medicine. Men, half of them bearded, outnumbered women two to one, and everyone was informally dressed. People seemed to know one another and the talk was lively. Between greetings to friends Bill explained the format of this Third Annual Master's Class.

George, he said, had been furnished a written digest of the case to be considered. After studying it briefly he had met with the patient and her doctor in a room across the hall to take the case on closed circuit television. Now he would join us to analyze the case while running the TV tape, stopping it periodically to explain his thoughts and ask the class questions. The audience would try to name the correct remedy before George finally revealed it.

"He'll do his best," Bill assured me, "to mislead us and conceal his solution until the last possible moment. He loves to mystify, but all the time he's grudgingly giving clues. He makes it into a game, and everybody loves it. He's such a good showman, it's easy to overlook his brilliance. In England last month, he got spectacular results in 48 out of 50 tough cases—and the other two responded when they switched pharmacies. The man's incredible. There's been no one like him for a hundred years!"

A BBC cameraman with a Beatle haircut and earrings was swinging his camera to make sure it would cover the two big TV screens on either end of the low stage. While final electronic adjustments were being made, Dr. Roger Morrison, told us George was avidly sought as a homeopathic lecturer in Norway, China, Belgium, New Zealand, Holland, Israel, Australia—in fact everywhere that homeopathy flourished. Ready now to begin, Roger looked around the room for the Greek master.

Out of the corner of my eye I saw the bright-eyed man by the Swiss lady stand up and take off his tan windbreaker. Walking down the aisle, he was greeted with thunderous applause. On stage he stood beaming, head tipped back, rocking sideways back and forth, a trim youthful man in a tan dress shirt and a dark brown tie that matched his slacks. Grey sideburns framed a handsome tan smiling face beneath closecropped dark hair. I knew he was 54, ten years older than Bill, but he didn't look it.

When the applause died away, George plunged without preamble into one of the homeopath's thorniest dilemmas: when to wait after giving a remedy and when to prescribe again. He spoke excellent English with a gallic accent and a foreigner's phraseology. "The patient may say, 'I get no effect, no result,'" he shrugged expressively. "He wants something more, but you wait because you see something he does not. There is movement. Sometimes I wait two ... four ... six months when the patient sees no change. Other times the patient imagines improvement, but I do not see it. He is trying too hard to help me.

"This time I do not wait. The remedy is not working, so I retake the case and give him something else. Or, if the remedy seems right, I try another pharmacy. Who knows if the first remedy was any good?" Another shrug. "When we take a case we must listen to the heart, recognize the ego and look beneath the words." He put a finger to one ear. "What we hear must be more than what the patient says!" Turning to the blackboard behind him, he drew profiles (wavy lines) to depict his four groupings of cases. Group A patients got one line, reflecting the fact that a single constitutional remedy ran through their entire lives.

"These people," he explained, "you find in untouched civilizations ... remote parts of Brazil and Peru. They are untouched by drugs of either kind. That's the main difference. In these places, homeopathy is most effective. We make miracles. With these simple people we are heroes, eh? Cancer is rare but in this group we can cure it. In South America, 25% of the people are in group A. In America, only 6%. Here you have too many drugs. Not enough emotion! You Americans are too controlled. You don't know how to cry." He waved a scolding finger at the audience.

"Group B patients," he went on, "require at least two remedies. They are twice as hard to cure because you have to be right twice." He tapped his forehead for emphasis. "After the first remedy works, you must find the second—and not give it too soon. The second remedy picture is always less apparent ... more subtle. Be careful! It is easier to go wrong than before!" Group C people, he explained, needed at least three remedies, and Group D patients required more than four. "This is what you find in New York. Too much civilization!" He shook his head reprovingly.

"Remember, these are just my ideas. You must seek others. For me there are not just three miasmas. I respect the people who say only three, but I do not agree. Today, we find a drug layer in many people. Often we must first treat for penicillin poisoning, or cortisone or marijuana, before we give a constitutional remedy. You are going to find confusion if you don't know this theory."

"Right on!" muttered Bill.

"And don't be upset by a sudden outbreak of asthma or arthritis in the patient you've been sucessfully treating for three years of schizophrenia. 'What the hell have I been doing?' you ask yourself."

144

Dramatically he hit his forehead with the heel of his hand. "But do not forget, the new symptoms are on the surface, so there hasn't been a setback after all. Never forget: from inside to outside, from above ... down. That signifies progress. It's the same when the patient stops coming. It's a good thing when the homeopath loses his patient." He paused, waiting to see if his meaning was understood.

"To make room for his family and friends," quipped a voice from the audience, provoking general laughter.

"Yes!" he nodded, smiling. Having completed the preliminaries, George waved the cameraman to begin. The TV screens came to life and we saw Nancy Herrick, P.A. (Physician's Assistant) in a room much like ours, explaining her case to George. Both were seated in folding chairs, and an empty chair stood between them. An attractive blond woman in her thirties, Nancy impressed me with her sympathy for the patient and her concise, articulate presentation. I knew she was a Hahnemann homeopath and Roger's wife.

"Is she good?" I asked Bill.

"She's *damn* good!"

The patient, Nancy explained, was a thirty-three year old woman who had first come to Hahnemann for treatment a year and a half before. Jane (as we'll call her) was suffering from chronic hepatitis contracted six years before from a blood transfusion. She was chronically tired, depressed and thirsty for alcohol. After taking her case, Nancy gave Natrum sulphuricum (Nat sulph) which produced dramatic improvement. But six months later Jane developed horrible vaginitis with an odor so putrid and penetrating that she refused to go out in public.

Nancy gave her a solution of Calendula and Chamomilla to treat it. It helped the vaginitis but antidoted the Nat sulph, bringing Jane renewed grief, deep depression, irritability, insomnia and suicidal thoughts. And she failed to respond immediately to stronger doses of Nat sulph. She divorced her husband and admitted to cruelly driving away the lover who succeeded him.

"Antidoting with something that mild means a low vital force," Bill whispered. Over the next year, Nancy saw Jane half a dozen times and tried several other remedies without effect. At one point

Jane went back to her allopath, but a D & C and various high pow-ered drugs brought no relief, so she returned to homeopathy—the only thing that had helped her.

George waved for the tape to be stopped. "This case illustrates the difficulty of finding the second remedy," he pointed out. "Here we see a woman who fights a lot. She shows us a weak vital force and a strong system, but her defenses are weak. There may be something quite malignant working here." He waved to the cam-eraman and Nancy resumed talking.

At present Jane was suffering from severe hemorrhage, fatigue, depression, feelings of impending doom and fear of people hurting her. Other symptoms included: poor energy, cravings for sugar and cold water instead of alcohol, and manic tendencies, with periods of frantic activity alternating with apathy. The only good news was improved abdominal symptoms after the last dose of Nat sulph— and a willingness to let George take her case.

"But she's a different person every time I see her," Nancy said helplessly. "I don't know what to do next." Her presentation com-plete, she looked hopefully at George.

The Greek master nodded. "The vaginitis could lead to cancer, of course. I first try to order the information in my mind. I ask myself, 'Was the first remedy correct?' For now I will assume 'yes.' What else do we know? The Chamomilla caused a relapse. She does not now want alcohol, so the liver is better. Nat sulph *has* acted, but what next?" He shrugged. "This case belongs to group C or D. There are surely more remedies underneath. I must try to find the second one. But does the liver need more help, first? Something deep we don't know about has happened to this woman to make her react so strongly. Something emotional, I think. Something traumatic. We must try to find out what. . . . These are my thoughts as I am about to meet her."

He sighed and smiled at Nancy. "All right, bring her in." On the screen we watched an impeccably dressed, unusually beautiful, completely composed young woman seat herself daintily in the vacant chair and confidently smile at Nancy and George. Her com-posure, sophistication and beauty came as a shock after what we had heard. But when the camera zoomed in on her movie star face, the shock was even greater. Her large hypnotic dark eyes made me shudder with a feeling I couldn't name. And I wasn't alone. Gasps and murmurs buzzed through the room.

George froze the closeup on the screen and asked us, "What do you see in those eyes?" I saw an unnerving intensity. Others in the audience called out, "Anger," "Wariness," "Deceit," "Protective-ness," "Aggressivness," and Bill said, "Fear." Ignoring the comments, George said, "Again I say, something traumatic has happened. I see it in her eyes. We must find out what it is."

The closeup of Jane's haunting eyes receded as the tape began again. George began by asking innocuous questions, using his charm, building Jane's confidence, confirming nonetheless a good many of Nancy's observations. At first Jane seemed confident and composed, but gradually she confirmed every one of the symptoms Nancy had reported, blushing slightly, occasionally ducking her head with embarrassment.

George again stopped the tape. "What I do," he told us, live, "is not mathematics and not fantasy either. I see fear and hear depression. Too much. Now we are ready. I will ask the central question, 'Why?'" When the tape began again we heard him ask Jane kindly, "The depression you speak of, have you always had it? When did it start? Can you remember?"

"In my late teens."

"Did it start with some event?"

Jane hesitated. "Primarily with a rape," she said smoothly.

"I see. You were raped. By a relative or close friend?" His tone was casual and friendly.

"A boy I knew back in high school … a friend. He was three or four years older. He'd come back from Vietnam … changed. He simply wouldn't let me alone."

"Was there a gun? Did you fear for your life?"

She nodded, wiping her eyes.

George stopped the tape and spoke to us. "There was a gun and she was raped. It affected her deeply. This is what we have been looking for … the emotional trauma that upset her system." When the tape resumed we learned that the Vietnam vet claimed to love her and wanted her to go away with him. When she gently

147

refused, he began to harrass her, following her everywhere, shouting at her, hitting her, waiting outside the house where she lived with her parents. "The stalking and threatening and terrorizing made my life a nightmare," she said calmly. "I felt terribly guilty."

"Guilty? Why guilty?" George asked sharply.

"My parents gave me no support. They believed I'd done something to encourage his behavior ... broken a promise, something like that. They were convinced I was attracting him, promoting his actions. They gave me no sympathy at all. I was angry at them because they didn't believe me. And because they seemed to think I was a ... tramp."

"How did the rape occur?" George urged. "Tell me what happened." She had gone, she told him, to a Frosty stand with friends for ice cream. When her friends left, the man had come up behind her with a gun and forced her to get into his car. After driving her into secluded woods, he threatened to kill her if she resisted. Then he raped her in an old abandoned church.

"Did you tell your parents?" George asked.

"No, I never spoke of it." She hung her head.

"Why not?"

"I guess I felt too ashamed. Since they believed I was at fault, I guess I did, too. I'm pretty sure they would have condemned me if I'd told them. So I didn't."

"Never?"

"No, never." She lowered her eyes.

George stopped the tape to tell us, "I need to know about her guilt because I'm thinking about Ignatia and Natrum mur. It is clear to me that she was paralyzed with fear by the rape. It broke her control. But she kept it inside. She never expressed it, so it weakened her body."

Bill had been writing furiously all the while. Now he leaned back and nodded. "We see that kind of thing all the time," he whispered, "physical symptoms following great emotional stress."

When the tape came back on George was asking Jane how she felt afterwards. She said her life had stopped. She didn't want to live. George nodded and asked about her parents and their background. We learned she was half Cherokee Indian and her parents were highly moralistic rigid people.

"So you never told them what happened. Did you tell anybody?" he prodded.

"I finally told my husband . . . just last year."

"It happened fifteen years ago and you never told anyone until last year?"

She nodded, looking embarrassed.

George nodded sympathetically.

"Do you hate men?" he asked suddenly.

She was caught off guard. "Um . . . no. Not really. But maybe I don't trust them. . . ."

"Because one hurt you?"

She nodded.

"Do you hurt them now?" he prodded. "To get back at them? Or maybe to protect yourself?"

"No, I don't think so." Her voice was cool and controlled again. Nancy had told us in detail how mean and cruel Jane had been, by her own admission, to both her husband and more recently to her lover. But she apparently wasn't prepared to admit it now to the unknown audience behind the camera.

"You don't get even a little sulky?" George wheedled.

"Yes . . . I guess I do." She seemed embarrassed.

The Greek master nodded, apparently satisfied. The tape stopped, and the George on the stage addressed us. "Now I have the whole picture," he declared, bouncing on his toes. "Her loathing of life, caused by the rape at age eighteen, brought on the hepatitis many years later. She was paralyzed by fright. So look up in your books, 'Ailments from Fright.'" There was a sound of fluttering pages as the audience bent over its reference books.

"We find secretiveness and silent grief, which makes us think of Ipecac and Natrum mur," the master observed. Again the pages rustled. Beside me, Bill flipped swiftly through his books, as eager as any of his students to find the answer first. "But does she like slimy foods? We don't know!" he muttered to himself.

"Is this Natrum mur?" George asked, shrugging. "No, it cannot be. We must resist the temptation," he answered himself. "Do you think she is 'cutoff'?" Half the audience raised hands in assent. George nodded noncommitally and strode thoughtfully across the stage. "Is this silent grief we see?" he asked, "or forced silence? The difference here is big. Is she silent because she fears her father will kill the boy and get in trouble if she tells him? In other words, is she silent to keep her father out of prison?"

He looked inquiringly at his rapt audience before continuing. "We must ask ourselves, How did she feel? Frightened? Nervous? Is this free-floating anxiety? Or impending doom? Or disaster?" I watched Bill madly flip the well-worn pages and scribble notes. Each of George's familiar phrases, I was surprised to discover, was a completely separate category in Bill's *Repertory*. These slight distinctions, I now saw, were important. The remedy pictures noted under each were substantially different—at least in the matter of degree.

Meanwhile, George was observing, "We see she doesn't fight against crying, the way a Natrum mur would. She even laughs while she talks. So it's not just anxiety. It's 'Fear of the Future.' Or 'Something Bad Will Happen.'"

"Are those really different?" I whispered to Bill.

He nodded, flipping the pages with practiced speed to show me separate categories under those apparently synonymous headings. "I'm predicting Arsenicum," he said, clearly caught up in the chase. "But Phosphorus is a close second."

George was beaming now at the consternation on the faces before him. "We must consider Natrum sulphuricum because it helped her once," he reminded his audience. "Remember, her blood is bright red with black dots. The smell is putrid and permeates everything." His tone was clinical.

Bill leaned my way. "We have to use our repertories, but he does all this out of his head," he said admiringly. "The judgements are subtle, but he's rarely wrong. Now he'll start looking for keynotes," he predicted.

"Has he a photographic memory?" I asked.

"No, just exceptional concentration."

"We could give her Phosphorus," George mused, scratching

his head, "but the putrid blood clots don't fit. Is she thirsty? Warm or cold? How exactly does she handle anxiety?"

"Now he's checking Pulsatilla. I'd never have thought of that!" Bill shook his head in wonder.

George switched on the tape and once again we watched him talking to Jane. The stage was now set for the denouement. With deft and rapid questioning, George eliminated Jane's fear of poverty and her tendency to express anxiety through hyperventilation. He determined that she was not restless and her time of best energy was early evening. Now Bill could hardly stay in his chair. He was bouncing up and down as the suspense mounted, flipping wildly through his books. "He's driving me crazy!" he said happily.

On the screens, in response to George's inquiries, Jane reported a bloated feeling in her stomach that was worse with cold. The master stopped the tape to hint at Carbo vegetablis, followed by Sulphur. When he mentioned Medorrhinum, Bill groaned, "He plays with us and teases, but it forces us to think."

George glanced at his watch. "I try to eliminate remedies by finding her main state. Will she confirm Carbo veg by revealing a main feeling that is 'Indifferent to Everything?' We will see after dinner." Without further comment, he stepped off the stage and commenced talking to the people who quickly crowded around him.

"He loves to leave us dangling," Bill smiled. He reached in his briefcase and brought out a two-inch Sony TV, which he set up on its stand and tuned to the fourth game of the World Series. The Mets were trying to even it at two games each with Boston at Fenway Park, and Bill had bets on the Mets with three or four members of the audience, including Michael. Within moments a group was clustered around Bill and his set. George and Jane and the mystery were temporarily forgotten.

When we returned to the conference room after dinner, Bill turned on his TV while the cameraman completed preparations. The Mets were leading 5–1 in the seventh. The set snapped off when the television monitors on stage came to life and George strolled up to stand between them. His tie was missing and his shirt was now open at the throat.

"So," he began. "Let us see how many keynotes we have, so

far." He counted on his fingers. "She sleeps on her right side and cannot sleep on the left. That pushes me toward Phosphorus but I don't jump—not yet. I may come back to it, but right now I probe for Medorrhinum."

He waved for the tape to begin. On the screens he asked Jane, "Your feet are cold, yes?"

"No, they're warm."

"What kind of fruits do you like best?"

"Strawberries and bananas."

"Do you ever go to the sea for vacation?"

"Yes, I love the sea."

George stopped the tape to comment, "She likes the sea, but not the right fruits. We were hoping for oranges or apples ... something sour. I want one more keynote, but I do not get it. Her feet are not cold. Where does that leave us?" He looked inquiringly at the audience, eyebrows raised. Various hesitant comments rose from the crowd, but he ignored them. "I like to see strong keynotes, but we must not lose sight of the patient's personality type, the clue to her essence. Is she volatile, passionate, sexual, extroverted, exploding? No, not her. Let's go back to the interview."

When the TV tape resumed, we saw George asking Jane about the workings of her mind. She complained that her thoughts were fuzzy and she had difficulty verbalizing. I thought she seemed unusually articulate, but George passed over her answer to ask her to name her biggest fear.

"Losing my job. I'm a systems analyst." When George looked baffled she added, "I work with computers."

"Are your nails strong?" he asked, taking one of her hands and examining the back, then turning it over. He stopped the tape. "Why do I look at her hand?" he asked the class. "Am I a palmist? Do I check for sweat? No, I look for redness in the palm, an indication of late stage liver disease. It is there. Do you notice her hands are gripping tightly together in her lap. She looks calm but is tightly controlled in her emotions. I find her very American, highly controlled and disciplined."

"He's forgotten Medorrhinum," Bill leaned over to whisper. "He's hunting Phosphorus again."

The tape was running again and we saw George asking how long she'd been divorced.

"Three years."

"But you've had lovers since then?"

When she nodded he went on, "Have you a sexual relationship now?"

Blushing, eyes downcast, she nodded again.

"Then you're not holding back? Do you have orgasms?"

"I don't think I hold back, but sometimes I feel timid. And sometimes I fake orgasms."

"But you feel an inclination to be attached?"

"Oh, yes."

"Is your relationship mostly sexual, or has it also been emotional? Do you talk with your lover about your feelings?"

"Recently, yes, it's been emotional, too."

George stopped the tape to comment. "We know she has anxiety about her parents, with strong guilt. She is sexually open but not sensual. That fits Phosphorus. And Phosphorus likes emotional commitment. Despite the rape, she can have sex, mostly with orgasms. Is she closed or open?"

The chorus from the floor said, "closed."

Bill turned to me. "Open or closed. That's a basic classification among the major remedies." The tape was running again, and George was asking, "Are you afraid of the dark?" Murmurs rose from the audience as knowledgeable homeopaths recognized a shift in the line of questioning. It was leading to the confirmtion or denial of a well-known keynote.

"Yes!" Jane said with feeling. "As a teenager I couldn't sleep in a dark room. I had to have the light on or I couldn't go to sleep."

"What were you afraid of? The dark itself? Ghosts? Men? Or something coming?"

"Something coming! That's it!"

Bill nudged me to point out a category in his *Repertory* entitled, 'Something Coming.' "She's a perfect Phosphorus!" he hissed. "Her imagination *creates* her fear."

Meanwhile on the TV screens Jane was volunteering that train whistles in the night scared her. So did thunder.

153

"Do you socialize easily?" George asked her.

"Not right now, I don't."

George stopped the tape to observe, "Phosphorus has a natural openness, but that may be contradicted when the person has been highly stressed and becomes fragile and vulnerable as a result." For the last time he started the tape and we saw him asking Jane if she'd ever taken hallucinogenic drugs.

"Only once." she blushed. "I think it was mescaline."

"And what happened?"

"It was terrible! Like a nightmare! Six foot high rats were shooting rockets at me! Never again."

George got up and went to her, taking her hand. "You didn't do anything bad," he said gently. "But you *are* too controlled. The rape affected you deeply."

She nodded, with a quick laugh that turned to a sob. She ducked her head to hide tears, wiping her eyes.

George put a comforting hand on her shoulder. "Don't try to stop yourself," he urged. "Crying is the best outlet. Tears are a very good release, a natural way of expressing emotion. We need to be expressive or we destroy the body. Your emotions are part of you, alive and intense. You don't want to stifle them."

She patted her eyes, her head still hanging, but clearly she felt better. "I know," her voice quavered, "but crying makes me feel weird."

"That's because you're not used to it. It makes you feel guilty. In America it is good to laugh but bad to cry." He shrugged helplessly. "I don't understand it. It's not natural. And it makes many problems." He patted her shoulder, smiling. "Try to cry when you feel bad," he said gently. "It will make you feel good."

The tape ended with George sitting close beside Jane, talking to her quietly, holding her hand. On stage now, he delivered a summary of the case. He seemed as vibrant and youthful as when he began three hours before. "What do we have?" he asked, bouncing on his toes, counting on his fingers. "Liver trouble, thirst, hemorrhaging. Only Phosphorus answers that. She has free-floating anxiety about her job, her future, her parents. She cares deeply about her family—to the point of guilt. She didn't tell them about the rape in order to save them."

Bill raised a hand. "She didn't exactly say that, did she?" he asked his teacher.

"No, but I conclude it. I'll ask her to confirm it in the follow-up." He resumed his dissertation with a rhetorical question. "Should putrid menses take us away from Phosphorus? No. They merely hint that we might follow with Carbo veg. And maybe way down the line, Medorrhinum."

"Why Carbo veg?" Bill asked.

"In case the bloatedness is not handled by the Phosphorus. Worse in the morning also does not exclude Phosphorus. She's undergoing cirrhosis of the liver, as we deduce from the hepatitis. Finally, the picture is clear. Phosphorus must work for her. I gave her Phosphorus 200. In a month we'll do a follow-up, just before I leave, to see what it does for her."

Bill asked, "How do you rate her curability?"

George shrugged. "She has a weak vital force, as shown by the antidoting of gentle Calendula. I have tried in every way to establish the best remedy. I am well satisfied with Phosphorus. But who knows. We shall see."

One of Bill's students, who had been holding up his hand for some time, received a nod from the master. "Would Phosphorus have worked in the beginning?" he asked respectfully.

"No ... well maybe just a little. The picture was different then. Nancy was right to give Natrum sulphuricum. It took off a layer and changed the picture to what we now see. If the Phosphorus does not work, we have good grounds to think of Carbo veg. We have done all we can. Now it is time to wait and see what Phosphorus can do."

He bowed slightly. The first case of the Master's Class was over. As applause filled the room he stood beaming above the crowd, soaking up the adulation, swaying slightly, restless hands playing with the microphone cord. When Bill stood up, others rose, and soon the entire audience was standing and clapping. Then the applause died away and Bill's miniature TV set was broadcasting the postgame wrapup. The Mets had won 6–2. Michael and the others crowded close, wallets out.

Suddenly George's face appeared in their midst. "So!" he nodded sardonically. "This is my competition!" He leaned close to peer briefly at the tiny screen. Then he smiled and walked away. The homeopaths looked like naughty boys.

When the others had departed, Bill said, "I've been wondering what to get him to take home to Greece. He folded the little set and put it back in his briefcase. "He'll enjoy one of these. He loves electronic gadgets."

Follow-Up on Jane

A month later, before returning to Greece, George did his follow-up. When he asked Jane, "How are you better?" she giggled uncharacteristically.

"The changes are mostly emotional," she told him. "I'm not afraid anymore. I go out now in public and take part in group activities. My fatigue is gone and I'm taking dance classes again. I'm much happier now, but my appetite is so good that I'm putting on weight."

Her memory had improved, the nightmares had stopped, her menses had normalized and her anxiety and depression were greatly lessened.

At last report, Jane was soon to be married.

11

Homeopathic Potpourri

My Isopathic Report ... Pharmacist Michael Quinn ...
Improved Eyesight ... Breakthrough Research ... Treating
Dying Dogs ... Dr. Deanne's Seven Cases ... My
"Breakdown" ... Allopathy Indicted

Before returning to watch George again, I sat down with Bill to report on the isopathic remedy. "I'm glad it helped," he grumbled, "but I don't like isopathics because they're suppressive. In that respect they're not really homeopathic, but I figure you can handle the suppression because your vital force is so strong."

I gave him a brief account of Dave Lund's work with the low speed drill. He was pleased—but not surprised—to hear that the nerve had resisted infection. Homeopathy had probably made the difference.

"And you didn't notice any ... ah. ... You didn't antidote?"

I smiled at his delicacy. "Only the isopathic. You said my attitude toward cats and bacon would change if I lost the Tuberculinum ... and they didn't."

He nodded. "You'd be a lot more irritable, too. Looks like you got away with it, thanks to your strong constutition. Maybe I'll experiment with low speed drills with other patients, since all dentists have them for cleaning."

"So, what do you think is happening to me?"

"I really can't explain it. The Tuberculinum shouldn't have survived all those antibiotics last winter. They're a pretty universal antidote. But I can't deny all the progress you've made. *Something's* sure working. Maybe the antibiotics cured you!" He chuckled at his joke.

I asked him why my aggravations had dramatically vanished in Hawaii, along with the fungus, only to bounce back intact a few weeks later.

"That's something I *can* explain. When there's an acute siege like you had, your vital force withdraws its energy from fighting the chronic condition in order to attack the more threatening acute condition. That's why your skin eruptions suddenly got better. Then as soon as the acute was cured, energy was focused again on the chronic problem, bringing back your aggravations.

"So there's nothing to do constitutionally, right?"

"Nope. Just have fun in Hawaii." He looked at his watch. "We just have time for lunch before the afternoon session."

That night, walking back to the Clinic with Bill, I asked his advice for my eighty-year old mother. She'd just told me, her voice breaking, that she'd been diagnosed as having cancer of the uterus. Her allopaths at Kaiser Hospital wanted to give her an immediate hysterectomy. I pleaded with her to get a second opinion—ideally from Bill. She said I could ask him. I feared that, like most doctors, he wouldn't venture an opinion without examining her. I was wrong. He said, "Tell her to go ahead with the hysterectomy."

"Really? Can't homeopathy help?"

"Sure, but with her age, her medical orientation and all the drugs she's taken, it would be much too slow. The surgery is routine and shouldn't be too hard on her, even at her age." I felt relieved. Suddenly we had our second opinion—and it came from the man I trusted most.

At the Clinic the light was still on in Michael's Pharmacy, though it was past ten o'clock on a Friday evening. The sandy-haired pharmacist was checking out his new machine. I stayed to inspect the strange contraption on which I'd become so dependent. The Skinner machine he'd ordered had never become available, so he designed his own and had it built. It sat on a butcher-block table in a brilliantly lighted white cubicle whose air was continually being filtered to protect against contamination. The machine looked like something Rube Goldberg might have dreamed up for NASA.

My isopathic remedies, said Michael, were the first two high potency concoctions prepared on this whirring, clanking, ratcheting machine. When I thought of him sitting here watching bleary-eyed in the middle of the night to make sure nothing went wrong—after a full day's work—I understood why Bill had said, "I admire the hell out of that man. He'll make any sacrifice for homeopathy."

Since it isn't known whether succussion (pounding) is more energizing than fluxion (violent mixing) in the preparation of high potency remedies, Michael's machine provides both. But the pharmacist is convinced that succussion is the key to maximum potency. His belief is rooted in copius research (e.g. Lampson) showing that it's the water, not the remedy, that carries the vital characteristics of the medicine when succussion accompanies dilution.

Fresh evidence of this contention surfaced in the summer of 1988 when the prestigious British scientific journal *Nature* published research results from scientists working independently in France, Italy, Israel and Canada. All four laboratories found that microdoses of medicine CAN have a therapeutic effect, even though they no longer contain even a single molecule of the original substance.

This so threatened orthodox medicine that a flying squad of ghostbusters and professional debunkers was sent out to discredit the results. After all, the researchers had broken the rules by contradicting revered scientific beliefs dating back two centuries.

Under this bombardment, *Nature* caved in and published a retraction, but when the smoke had cleared the results were grudingly accepted by open-minded scientists everywhere. The research was a breakthrough of sorts for homeopathy. Here was scrupulous and independent laboratory confirmation of what homeopaths had consistently observed for two hundred years: as long as a solution is vigorously agitated (i.e. successed) each time it's diluted, its potency remains despite the absence of any vestige of the original substance.

So apparently a substance leaves its imprint on the molecular structure of the diluting water long after the original substance is gone. This largely explains the well-documented process of potentization that homeopaths have relied on for nearly 200 years.

Michael discovered homeopathy while still an undergraduate at the University of Wisconsin in the early 1970's. Its impact was profound. "I felt a personal resonance with homeopathy," he told me. "Here was a cause with a scientific basis where my talents could make a difference to mankind. It was just what I'd been looking for." After obtaining a degree in pharmacy he set out in search of an almost nonexistent job as a homeopathic pharmacist. When he learned of the impending birth of Hahnemann Clinic, he came to Berkeley to ask Bill Gray for a job, determined to convince the Clinic's founders that they needed him.

To his surprise and delight Bill welcomed him warmly. The Clinic had been looking for a pharmacist and wondering how to find one. But before the job materialized, Hahnemann ran into organizational problems. Michael saw his dream slipping away. So he quit his high-paying pharmaceutical job and came to Berkeley to freely contribute his organizational skills and take over the struggling clinic's fouled up bookkeeping.

Finally, at Christmastime, 1984, the last obstacles were overcome. Michael telephoned an order to Bornemann in Philadelphia for a full complement of homeopathic remedies, and he spent the final week of the year painting his pharmacy, building furniture and putting up shelves. When the remedies arrived he was able, by working nights, to have Hahnemann Pharmacy ready to fill prescriptions when the Clinic opened for business on New Years Day, 1985. He's been there ever since, working hand in glove with the Clinic's physicians, doing everything necessary to meet the varied needs of its patients.

Back in Hawaii for our second winter, I was anxious at first about the devastating infections that had struck so quickly the year before. I vividly remembered the crotch rash that made me walk like Fred Sanford and the Elephant Man brow that scared little children. Twice a day I scrubbed vigorously in the shower and examined myself closely for the beginnings of rash. But the days turned to weeks and nothing happened.

Then, in December, I began to experience strange feelings of nausea while working at my word processor. At first it only happened when I'd been writing for some time or was tired. But it swiftly got worse until it started as soon as I sat down to work. Finally I realized it had something to do with the glasses I'd worn for reading for five years.

The next time we drove to Kona I visited the supermarket's ready-to-wear rack of "prescription" glasses. Borrowing a paperback with small print, I tried various pairs, starting with the lowest magnification and working up. The pair I selected let me read the fine print but didn't bring nausea. The magnification was 1.25—exactly half the 2.50 of the glasses I'd been using!

When I took them home, the problem vanished! A year and a half earlier I had been skeptical when Bill told me homeopathy should improve my eyesight. Now it had happened! I soon found I could work at the computer without glasses at all, and I could read the newspaper and most books—so long as I sat in the natural light on our screened-in lanai.

The return to Hawaii, after six months away, provided a fresh perspective on my overall condition, just as it had at the cabin four months earlier. And the comparison pleased me just as much. I now found myself remarkably philosophical about the inescapable din in our village, which had often irritated me in the past. We could still hear our neighbors' stereos, crying kids, cars, domestic battles and TVs, but now they hardly bothered me.

I likewise found myself less likely to get mad at Deanne or Gellie. Ever since my passage through primal therapy I had been highly expressive of all kinds of feeling. I blew up briefly when something angered or frustrated me. And I laughed and expressed joy just as readily. This winter there was distinctly more laughter than anger.

One January day my friend Brian Nelson told me his beloved Makua, a tiny female Chihuahua, was dying of heart worms. The vet had told him the standard treatment of arsenic killed substantially more pets than it cured. "I can't stand to watch her slowly die of heartworms," he said unhappily, "but I can't bring myself to let the vet kill her with arsenic, either. She coughs all the time and she's getting pretty feeble. I don't know what to do."

The vet had explained that not only was it necessary to kill the heartworms without fatally poisoning the dog, it was vital to do it slowly so the dead worms could be assimilated. Kill them too fast and they would kill the dog by clogging veins and arteries. Brian's partner Al also had a dog dying of heartworms. It seemed to be a common problem on the island.

I suggested he try a homeopathic vet and gave him Michael Traub's phone number. Michael referred him to Richard Pitcairn, DVM, the renowed homeopathic vet in Portland, Oregon, who in turn referred him to Dr. Deva Kaur Khalsa, DVM, in Pennsylvania. When Brian called her she told him she'd cured at least twenty cases of heartworm homeopathically and had never lost a patient. She promised to send Brian the remedy, and she did.

A week later he called us, guardedly optimistic.

"Her instructions say the medicine contains Arsenic, but acts very slowly. It may be six months before all the worms and eggs are dead. I don't care how long it takes, if it works. I give it to Makua in her food twice a day. Al does the same with Moa. Dr. Khalsa said there ought to be signs of improvement within a month."

Our return to Hawaii also revealed my changed attitude toward competition. Every evening before sunset I drove down to Spencer Beach Park to play basketball with the locals. After a friend got me on the Mauna Kea Beach Hotel's spare tennis player list I was often called to play singles or fill out a doubles foursome. An elderly gentleman named Bill asked me to be his regular bridge partner in the island's duplicate tournaments. After several games I told him, "Bill, I can't do this anymore. It just isn't fun!"

To a lesser degree it was the same with basketball and tennis. A few years before I had thrived on competition, getting high on winning ... and upset by defeat. Now I found myself ducking games with overly intense, aggressive players. I found I simply didn't enjoy them anymore. Games, I dimly remembered, were supposed to be fun! I no longer needed to compete—or win. To integrate my changed attitude, I developed a new set of priorities.

Having fun came first, not getting hurt was second, and winning ran a distant third. On the courts I found myself clowning and bantering and genuinely playful. Relaxed and having fun, I found I played better and won just as often!

Deanne had been radiantly healthy for nine months—dating back to her constitutional with Bill Gray. Then her old symptoms returned in November, especially when she drove up the mountain to cool and rainy Waimea to teach. By Christmas she had a nagging cough and complained of constant drainage down the back of her throat. At times her voice was so hoarse she could hardly make herself heard in the classroom. When two weeks of vacation from school failed to help, I urged her to consult Michael Traub. He suggested she first call Bill Gray.

We made it a mini-conference call, with Deanne on the office phone, me in the bedroom and Bill 2500 miles away in Berkeley. After a barrage of questions Bill told her she still sounded like classic Arsenicum, but suggested that Michael Traub retake her case to make sure. He guessed that the initial dose had worn off. If Michael found Arsenicum, Bill urged a single dose of a potency higher than the original 200.

Michael came a few days later to take Deanne's case. In the meantime, she remembered that Bill originally had had another remedy in mind if Arsenicum failed. But what was it? Deanne was sure it was somewhere in the computer. The three of us hunched over the screen trying disk after disk. Finally we found it. Bill's backup had been Silica. But after questioning Deanne closely Michael prescribed Arsenicum 1000, which he had thoughtfully brought with him.

For several weeks after taking the remedy, Deanne experienced aggravations in the form of intensified drainage. Then all her symptoms disappeared and she was once again healthy and happy. Throughout the winter in Hawaii, Dr. Deanne continued her successful acute prescribing. When someone we encountered complained about their health, she would deftly draw them out to classify the affliction. If it seemed acute and she thought she could help, she generously offered to take the case ... without charge.

Chronic problems were directed to Michael Traub or Hahnemann Clinic.

For instance, baby Matthew, who lived next door, got a quick dose of Hypericum when Deanne ran outside to find him screaming after smashing his finger in a car door. Within five minutes of treatment, his screams had subsided to a whimper.

Our daughter Gellie regularly got Calendula for cuts and scratches and for sunburn at the beach. Deanne gave her Aconite, Arsenicum or Pulsatilla for colds, and Hypericum and Arnica for frequent falls and bruises. Every day after school, or just before bed, she would present her various new playground wounds for treatment.

Our friend Winifred received Arnica to ease the pain of dental surgery, while Lynn across the street got Rhus tox for the back she strained playing tennis. Every time we took pale visitors from the mainland to the beach, we introduced them to soothing Calendula lotion for their inevitable sunburns.

One day an anxious lady named Debbie telephoned to tell us her sick baby boy badly needed Pulsatilla, but she couldn't make the fifty mile drive to Dr. Traub's office. Michael had suggested she call Deanne. Debbie arrived a few minutes later with her red-faced crying boy, bringing us a bag of dried fruit as a gift. Before she left we had made a new friend, and her baby boy, Jimmy, was peacefully sleeping in her arms. The Pulsatilla had already taken effect.

Glenn played clarinet in the combo that worked nightly at the nearby Mauna Kea Beach Hotel. We sometimes went there to dance on the terrace beneath the stars. And Glenn looked after our garden in the summer. One day he came to Deanne deeply worried. While hurrying to finish a gardening job he had severly pulled the ligaments in his left index finger. It was swollen to twice its normal size and he feared he might not be able to play the clarinet that night.

Deanne took his case and gave him Arnica. He came back the next day, smiling. Most of the swelling had quickly disappeared and he'd been able to play, but he still had some pain. Deanne gave him Ruta and the next time we saw him he flexed the healed finger, grinning. "No more pain or swelling," he reported. "But my girl-friend would like to talk to you about female problems."

A six year old named Jill, one of Gellie's playmates, seemed to have chronic earaches, so Deanne talked to her mother and gave her Mercury which brought quick relief. It always pains Deanne to hear that some child has been sick for a long period ... or living on Tylenol, antibiotics or aspirin. She tries hard to coax their parents into giving her permission to treat them. Almost half the time she's turned down out of ignorance or fear.

It's impossible to predict people's response to Deanne's offer of homeopathic help. Many an adult, whom we thought open and intelligent—and knew was in pain—has refused out of anxiety of some sort. "Oh, I'm not *that* bad!" they'll say, or "I'm allergic to herbs," or, "No thanks, I let my body heal itself." But other suffer-ers, who we judged to be timid, will say, "Sure, I'll give it a try." Every case is a fresh adventure.

For Christmas I ordered Deanne a set of seven tapes on acute pre-scribing by Dr. Ben Hole and Dana Ullman. They came from Dana's Homeopathic Educational Services (HES) in Berkeley, an admirable mail order source of books, tapes, kits, etc. (See "Home-opathic Sources, for HES's address.) The tapes were entitled "Inroduction to Homeopathy and How to Use a Home Medicine Kit." They proved to be excellent. Pen poised above her notebook, Deanne made notes as she listened. From time to time she would call me away from the computer to listen to some tidbit. Often enough I'd end up lying on the floor and listening to the end of the tape.

In January, someone stepped on my foot during a basketball game, wrenching my left achillies tendon. Deanne's quick dose of Arnica greatly reduced the pain, but I still limped. I was used to getting bumps and bruises on the court, and I was sure I'd be all right after a couple days rest. But I wasn't. As a teenager, my passion for high jumping had overly stretched my tendons. Ever since I'd had peri-odic flareups of tendonitis.

Now, to my dismay, I began to experience soreness in my right tendon, too! When I went to the court for my ritual evening game, sunset and swim, I often hobbled around like a decrepit old man for half an hour before my tendons were loose enough to run. When I got home I'd rub on Arnicated oil but it didn't help much.

Deanne consulted her reference books and proposed I take either Rhus tox or Ruta, which she had in her kit. I called Michael for his advice ... and to make sure neither would conflict with Tuberculinum. He recommended Ruta 6, assuring me it couldn't hurt since it wasn't a constitutional remedy. The Ruta brought overnight relief—every time I took it—but the tendonitis always came back.

I was wondering what to do when a bewildering series of afflictions struck in quick succession. Deanne later referred to them as my "breakdown." First came a fluke injury to my left kneecap, then a case of tennis elbow, then a bruise on the ball of my left foot, followed by a bone spur on my left thumb. I was president of the Village's homeowner association, but politics were new and strange to me, and I found myself anxious about conflicts within my board of directors. When I developed an itch on my right eyelid that grew inflamed, Michael told me to keep it clean and use Calendula. But it didn't get any better.

My friend Ken Kehoe, who had originally introduced me to homeopathy in that Death Valley swimming pool, arrived for a visit so sick with the flu that he could hardly walk. Deanne immediately took his case and gave him Gelsemium. Then we put him to bed on our lanai. The next morning he'd made a miraculous recovery. "I'm amazed!" he told us. "I feel ninety percent better!"

A day or so after he left I got chilled. The next day, not surprisngly, I came down with Ken's flu. Deanne went to work with her books and notes but she couldn't find a picture that stood out from the rest, so we made a conference call to Michael Traub. He proposed Lycopodium because the soreness in my throat had begun on the left side and was relieved equally well by either hot or cold liquids. Deanne gave me an immediate dose, and I took another just before sleep.

In the morning I felt marvelously improved, and by the time I went to bed that night I felt cured. So after five doses in 24 hours, I stopped the Lycopodium and resumed taking Ruta. Most prescribers, I remembered, urged stopping a remedy when improvement was great, so I felt I was doing the right thing. But two days later I had a relapse. When I called Michael he told me to get back on the Lycopodium and keep taking it until I was sure I was cured. "Stopping after marked improvement" did not apply, he said, to a heavy case of the flu.

When I told him I was running out of Ruta 6, he suggested I try Ruta 200. "Since we know it works, I think we're justified in giving a higher potency. One dose of 200 may be all you ever need."

The Lycopodium again brought immediate relief, but this time I didn't quit until a relapse seemed impossible. When I finally took the Ruta 200 it outlasted my multitude of muscular aches and pains. By the middle of March I was healthy. Even my anxiety about management of the village melted away after several harmonious board meetings. Only the itching in my right eyelid remained.

Then it dawned on me that it was worse after each application of Calendula. Could I possibly be allergic to this mildest of remedies? Could my body regard it as suppression? I quit and improvement was immediate! That must mean the Tuberculinum was still working. If I was right, it had worked its way back in time to my symptoms during adolescence—an impressive distance of some 40 years!

All I knew for sure was that this was my winter of acute remedies. One after another had brought me swift and impressive relief. It was almost worth suffering mild afflictions to see how wonderfully they could be cured by homeopathic remedies! Maybe the best way to win converts to homeopathy, as Dr. Linda Johnston says, is simply to treat the patient's bruises with Arnica and let them experience the miracle for themselves.

Arnica, Aconite, Calendula and Hypericum—for starters—should be prominently available wherever aspirin, antihistamines and Vaseline are sold!

In April, quite by chance, I happened to tune into two PBS television shows that provided some perspective on conventional medicine. The theme of the first was the familiar "Modern Medical

167

Miracles" and "Triumphs of Science," boasting about "impressive advances" in medicine.

Listening carefully I heard that every kind of human affliction is some kind of "disease." Nothing was ever said about the *causes* of these diseases. They just magically occurred. Advisedly the word "cure" was never used. (You could sue.) But a great deal was said about symptoms, those hateful manifestations of disease. They must be obliterated by any means ... at any cost to the patient's health or pocketbook. It was often "necessary" to poison the body with radiation or chemotherapy in the name of better health. It was likewise essential to surgically remove "abnormal" growths of any kind, since they were symptoms. If an organ didn't function well, rip it out.

It couldn't be helped if any of these treatments killed the patient, put him in the hospital or crippled him. The problem wasn't the drugs, it was the weakness of the patient. Side effects were simply unavoidable, and a small price to pay for the miracles of modern medicine!

The smooth-talking moderator in the pristine white coat never hinted that symptoms could represent simple degeneration or that the body might merely be manifesting internal imbalance. No sir! Symptoms meant disease! If the knee hurts, there's disease in the knee and we must do anything necessary to stop it from hurting, even if it creates worse pain elsewhere ... or later.

Your allopath will give you Cortisone and tell you proudly that he's "stopped" the disease in your knee. He won't talk about cause or prevention or the rest of your body or other symptoms or your mental or emotional health. Because he can't.... And this is what is meant by the "scientific" triumphs of modern medicine ... at a time in our history when America's health grows steadily worse! And the cost of health care rises a frightening 15% yearly.

The second program, on investments, analyzed the profit potential of pharmaceutical company stock for the coming year. An investment specialist for the drug industry told us pharmceutical companies spent $5 million in 1987 researching and developing new drugs. There were some "interesting" ones coming along ... with nice profit potential. None of them were cures and no "breakthroughs" were in sight, but some of the new drugs "ought to catch on." Despite the absence of cures, drug companies were highly profitable and the future looked bright for even greater earnings.

Research priorities, he told us, were drugs for AIDS, cancer, obesity, baldness, diabetes, high cholesterol, hypertension and arthritis. He bragged that researchers were making some headway in cutting down disastrous side effects. He defined a "truly exciting drug" as one which "actually produces some remission."

I couldn't help thinking what homeopathy could do with that $5 million for research. Nor could I help but compare Michael Quinn's night and day dedication to the production of inexpensive, effective high quality dilute remedies with the powerful, expensive, poorly tested offerings of the drug industry. Every business needs to make a profit to stay in business. It's ethics of operation that need to be examined. Consider the following. . . .

Consumer watchdog Ralph Nader's magazine Public Citizen in February, 1987, reported that America's pharmaceutical industry makes millions of dollars every year selling drugs that it *knows* do harm, using chemical components that have been *scientifically proven* to be harmful! And the FDA drags its feet on banning drugs proven to do harm or completely ineffectual.

For instance, said Public Citizen, Oraflex, an arthritic drug, killed more than fifty people before it was finally withdrawn. Selacryn caused serious liver damage and death among the hypertension victims who innocently took it on prescriptions from their physicians. Bendectin, for morning sickness, has been linked to serious birth defects. In each case, the producers of these drugs *knew* of the harm their medicines had done but did nothing until they were forced to!

"Remember that very special tingle in the leading mouthwashes a few years ago?" asks Public Citizen. "It was chloroform, a known carcinogen!" It took a lawsuit to get it banned. Pfizer, one of the pharmaceutical giants, introduced Feldene in April 1982. Since then, said Public Citizen, the FDA had received reports of 182 deaths and 2,621 adverse reactions to the drug. And still (at this writing) the drug has neither been withdrawn or banned!

These few examples tell you something about the motives and

ethics of the companies who supply the powerful, high priced, untested drugs that your family allopath unhesitatingly prescribes. Why does he prescribe them? Because the drug companies bankroll his medical schools, teaching hospitals and medical journals. His drawers are full of their free samples.

He's their "pusher." It's his job to prescribe the products they are hawking, although he may know nothing whatever about them —except what he's been told by the drug company salesman who brings the free samples and delivers the sales pitches developed in the high-powered marketing departments and advertising agencies. If these drugs do harm it's your fault for being allergic to them!

In late April we got a postcard from Ken Kehoe. Though he had introduced me to homeopathy and benefited from it greatly, he had admitted while visiting that he was suffering intermitantly from the Giardia he had picked up in the tropics a year before. Deanne had rekindled his enthusiasm for homeopathy by dramatically curing his flu overnight. Before he left he vowed to go straight to the Clinic to be constitutionally treated.

Ken's postcard reported that Roger Morrison had taken his case and given him China 200. If that wasn't working when he went back a month later, Roger planned to try Lycopodium.

Some months later Ken wrote, "China was close but not quite 'it.' I've been on Lycopodium now for six months, and improvements have been dramatic! I have more energy for work and play, a more positive outlook and vastly improved digestion and elimination. I'm 95% back to normal—for the first time in years. One of the biggest benefits is that I find myself more organized and responsible. That's a very positive change in my life."

Just before we returned to the mainland in May, we visited Brian Nelson and his dogs. When I remarked that bouncing, barking Makua seemed healthy, Brian grinned. "I think she's getting well, all right. I've been giving her the medicine for a couple of months. Her cough is gone and she's got back her vigor. Al's dog has done just as well. We're about to send stool samples to the vet to see if worms or their eggs are still present. We're not in any hurry. We'll keep giving our dogs medicine until we're sure they're cured."

The stool samples tested negative and both dogs have long been worm-free and healthy. "In fact," says Brian, "They're like puppies again. We're thrilled to have them back, and our vet plans to get the remedy we used."

12

Kids & Dogs Don't Lie!

The Homeopathic Education of Vet Richard H. Pitcairn, DVM ... Treating Dogs & Cats—Five Case Histories ... Ten Children's Cases From Michael Traub, ND and Peggy Chipkin, FNP

In its continuing effort to discredit homeopathy, the medical establishment never fails to attack the extreme dilution of homeopathic remedies, insisting that any benefit to the patient must be entirely "placebo response," i.e. imagined benefit from harmless inactive substances.

It's the patient's belief, they say, not the medicine, that causes improvement. It's "all in the patient's head," or the workings of faith or positive thinking. After all, it's been proven that as much as forty percent improvement may be explained by the placebo response.

But there can't be a placebo response from dogs and cats or preverbal children. They simply can't be "sold" or convinced. Since they can't understand the manner in which they're treated, they can't develop beneficial faith in that treatment. Therefore, marvelously effective homeopathic results achieved with seriously afflicted babies and pets, effectively refute the convenient accusations of allopathy.

Since these consistent and spectacular results may also help assure the reader of homeopathy's effectiveness, I want to present a modest sampling ...

172

Richard H. Pitcairn, DVM, Ph.D., is the premier homeopathic veterinarian in America, with a thriving Eugene, Oregon, practice known throughout the world. Because of his success, difficult cases are referred to him from everywhere. Since desperately sick animals can't easily jump on planes, he spends a good deal of time on the phone, consulting with other vets and anxious owners.

For instance, when our friend Brian's dog Makua was dying of heart worms in Hawaii, we urged him to call Naturopath Michael Traub, who in turn called Dr. Pitcairn in Eugene. Dr. Pitcairn referred him to yet another homeopathic vet, Dr. Deva Kaur Khalsa, who provided the curative remedies.

Back in 1978 Dr. Pitcairn was a conventional vet, searching among alternative methods of healing for a better way of treating animals. When he read George Vithoulkas' *The Science of Homeopathy*, it was the beginning of a journey. "That book meant a great deal to me," wrote Dr. Pitcairn. "After reading it, almost non-stop, I felt a great understanding fill me." With an unshakeable conviction that Hahnemann's healing art could work as well or better on animals than it did on humans, he tried to enroll in the International Foundation for Homeopathy's post graduate training program.

"My application was rejected because I was a veterinarian. It was felt at the time that a veterinarian could not really apply homeopathy in a constitutional or classical manner." (Thanks largely to Dr. Pitcairn's remarkable success, the IFH has reversed its policy and now welcomes vets.)

"That was a time of great frustration for me," he remembers. "But I felt intuitively that a way could be found to make homeopathy work for animals. I was thrown back on my own resources, but I was also free to experiment.

"There was some literature on the use of homeopathy in animals, but it did not satisfy my needs. It was mainly 'cookbook' suggestions for the treatment of a single symptom.

For instance, for diarrhea use Aloe, Arsencium album, Podophyllum or Veratrum album. That was all right for simple acute conditions, but what I saw in my practice in the majority of cases were symptoms caused by chronic or degenerative diseases. I wanted to be able to cure the most difficult diseases, like Kent describes in his *Lesser Writings*.

"I went to work in earnest, studying Kent, Hahnemann, Allen, Hering, Boger, Burnett and many other illustrious homeopaths. After years of self-study and experimentation, I finally developed effective methods—entirely from clinical experience—for applying homeopathy effectively to animals. I now exclusively use single remedies in both high and low potency. Classical homeopathy is what works best in my practice. Experience tells me I cannot achieve the same high quality results using more than one remedy, or alternating remedies, or combining allopathy with homeopathy.

"At first, following the cookbook suggestions, my treatments often produced little improvement or, at worst, aggravation of the original problem. Clearly, a way had to be found to apply the simillimum—the constitutional remedy. Since animals can't talk and report subjective symptoms, I had to develop a *new* method of eliciting information. It was like working with pre-verbal children. I had to treat the entire range of my patient's problems, but I could never talk to the patient!

"Except for the symptoms that could be seen physically, *all* my information had to come from the person closest to the animal.

"Another problem was that my materia medica only reported changes occurring in human beings. Would they be the same in detail for animals? Even if they were, how could one recognize, say, Arsenicum album, in a dog? Would there be the same restlessness and thirst? Would a cat be the same as a dog, or different? And what, above all, would be the major constitutional remedies for dogs and cats? Were they the same as in human beings? The same in each species? There was a lot to find out.

"But being a veterinarian I have two advantages over doctors who treat humans. I can treat serious conditions like cancers and severe infections, that, because of social pressures, would normally require hospitalization. And I am free to treat solely with homeopathic remedies, without pressure to use allopathic drugs.

"I gradually learned how to interview the person closest to the sick animal to elicit useful information. It involves substantial training of the client. With a human patient, one does not want to lead too much. We want the story to unfold in a natural way that reveals the patient's psyche. When working with an animal, however, the person being interviewed is merely an observer. To draw out reliable information, that person must be vigorously cross-examined like a witness in a trial.

"So I rigorously question and guide the discussion to get the information I need. I generally start by asking, 'What is the chief problem we are facing here?' When the client has covered the main points and begins to lose momentum, I go back to each of the major points and ask detailed, specific leading questions.

"For instance, I might ask, 'Does your dog lick its front feet excessively? If your dog has reduced appetite, is it usually the morning meal that he refuses?' (It usually is.)

"It often takes 45 to 60 minutes to go over the animal's history in this sort of detail. Some clients won't be able to answer accurately the first time around. If they seem unclear about some point, I ask them to be especially observant in that area next time because it has considerable importance for me. When I talk to them again they usually can tell me exactly what I need to know.

"And those observations must be free of gratuitous interpretation. For instance, a client recently told me her sick cat was now 'playing' with the other cat in the house.

"Rather than accept the word 'playing' as evidence that the patient was improving, I asked what she meant by 'playing?'

"'Well,' she replied, 'the other cat will suddenly run and jump on top of him (our patient) and then they roll around and wrestle.'

"Her more detailed answer now reveals that our patient is not playing at all. In fact, his condition has probably deteriorated, since the other cat, sensing his weakness, now takes advantage of the opportunity to dominate him.

"Often I ask my clients to keep a daily log, writing down what they observe so they won't forget anything. By repeatedly asking for certain information, I teach them to watch for it and become good observers. Once a remedy is decided on, I may tell the client,

'When you come in next time, I am going to ask you detailed questions about the following symptoms. Then I list them, urging the client to write them down.

"By using these stratagems, I have learned to elicit highly useful, reliable information, greatly reducing the obstacle of lack of direct communication. I have even discovered ways to get answers to questions from the animal itself. For instance, if I want to know if cold applications relieve symptoms, I ask the client to apply cold compresses on one occasion and warm ones on another. Then I ask them to closely observe the animal's reaction. Did one seem more welcomed than the other? It is surprising what the observing client can determine.

"If I suspect that the animal prefers warmth, I ask the client to put out a heating pad (on a low setting) to see if the cat gravitates toward it. If I wonder about the appeal of salty food, I ask that two plates be set out, one salted and the other not. We soon find out which the patient prefers. Since I cannot communciate verbally with the patient, I simply create situations that question non-verbally.

"Once the needed information is collected, my usual approach is to focus on the single most reliable physical or mental symptom and do a short eliminative analysis. Or sometimes a keynote will stand out and point to the needed remedy. Usually the constitutional remedy that emerges will be a polychrest—i.e. among the most frequently prescribed for humans. Unfortunately, many cases are so messed up by previous allopathic treatment and years of developing pathology, that the best I can do is treat step by step with a series of remedies, 'zig-zagging' to a cure.

"If there are too few objective symptoms available, I fall back on techniques I discovered in Hahnemann's *Organon*. Hahnemann suggests we make our best choice of remedy based on the single outstanding symptom that we have. This may mean picking the obvious polychrest—like Sulphur for itching skin. Then we watch very carefully for the patient's reaction. Maybe the remedy will be correct and the problem will be cured, but more likely the remedy will produce side effects.

"Hahnemann teaches us that these side effects also belong to the disease we are treating, even if they were undetectable before.

The first choice prescription, he tells us, may simply make the vital force respond and display the rest of the previously unperceived symptoms, so we can use them for our next prescription. The method works and I use it successfully all the time on animals.

"If there is no significant progress to a cure from the first remedy, I add the new symptoms—now more observable as a result of the treatment—to complete the disease picture. With this added information in hand, I can often make a second and more accurate prescription.

"Now let's look at an actual case to see how animals respond to homeopathy. Rocky was a 5-year old male Collie-Springer cross. Over the phone, I learned that a week before, after a bath, he suddenly became lame in his left shoulder, crying out in pain as he rose from the floor. The next day he could not rise at all and would neither eat nor drink. Movement of his head to the right caused intense pain. He was taken to an emergency clinic where an x-ray of his neck showed a 'slipped disc.'

"His past history of difficulty was not extensive. About a year before, his owner told me on the phone, Rocky started acting tired and stiff after the two of them jogged for several miles. And there were occasional itchy, inflamed 'hot spots' on his back. He didn't drink much water and he preferred the shade. Now he was lying very quietly without moving at all. When standing, his body was bent to the left.

"Since Rocky was clearly suffering and I wouldn't be able to see him for three days, I made a prescription over the phone—Bryonia 200c. I based my choice on the neck pain and Rocky's reluctance to move or turn his head.

"When I was able to examine him three days later, I found the Bryonia had helped temporarily, but then he had regressed and hadn't moved in the past 24 hours. Bryonia had been a reasonable guess, but not the right remedy.

"After making a careful examination and questioning Rocky's owner in detail, I characterized the case as follows: (1) the suddenness of the attack, (2) the violence of the symptoms, (3) the screaming from pain, (4) extensive inflammation of the muzzle, neck and abdomen; panting and acclerated heartbeat, (5) location of the pain in the neck, and (6) the painful reaction to moving the head.

"Using Kent's *Repertory* and the *Synthetic Repertory*, I found this combination pointed to Belladonna. I prescribed Belladonna 10M, to be given every four hours. After only two doses, Rocky startled his owner by running into the bedroom, asking to be let out. All in all, Rocky needed half a dozen doses over the next couple of weeks before he was cured. No other treatment has been needed during the past year. He now goes jogging with his owner, running with ease, and is completely recovered from his ordeal.

"This case clearly shows the superiority of homeopathic treatment over the allopathic alternative of dangerous and expensive drug therapy and spinal surgery. The quick response to the correct remedy is common in cases as sudden and severe as this one. If I hadn't seen strong improvement within 24 hours, I would have looked for another remedy without hesitation.

"Cases like this demonstrate that classical, constitutional treatment of animals is indeed possible. I regularly and successfully treat auto-immune diseases, skin allergies in dogs, deformative arthritis, chronic viral infections like Feline Leukemia, Feline Infectious Peritonitis, demodective mange and other severe skin problems, loss of appetite, cystitis, pavovirus, distemper, concussion, cancer, unresponsive anemia, chronic cystitis in cats, spinal disc herniation, punctures, gunshot wounds, diarrhea, depression, all sorts of personality problems, and other serious afflictions.

"Some of the methods I have learned to apply to animals should have value in the treatment of non-verbal children and adults who are so disturbed that they cannot communicate.

"It would be hard to explain cures like Rocky's as 'placebo effect' or the patient's 'imagination.' Thus treating animals homeopathically clearly demonstrates the dependable effectiveness of correctly prescribed homeopathic remedies.

"I once treated a cat suffering from a rare post-surgical reaction—septicemia. It was a crisis situation. Dark blood leaked from every orifice of her body and there was bleeding beneath the skin on her eyelids and ears. She got worse every moment and I was sure antibiotics wouldn't work fast enough to save her. While administering fluids into a vein, I noticed that she was hypersenti-tive to pain. That made me think of Arnica, so I gave it immediately.

"In a few hours she was greatly improved. I repeated the dose every few hours. The next morning her temperature was down and she no longer was bleeding. Soon she was much calmer, and eating for the first time in days. Within 48 hours of first receiving the Arnica, all that remained of that life-threatening situation were a few dry scabs. A week later she was as healthy as ever.

"As this acute case suggests, homeopathic medications gener-ally restore health more quickly than drugs.

"Another, older cat was shown by lab tests to be suffering from feline infectious peritonitis—a fatal condition not curable with con-ventional drugs. His symptoms included repeated vomiting, diarrhea, loss of appetite and swelling of the stomach. Over a period of days his owner and I switched him to a home-prepared diet and increased his vitality by the use of herbs and thymus gland supplement.

"In the process I came to recognize the symptom picture of Arsenicum album. When I gave it he experienced an aggravation of symptoms for several days, followed by continuous improvement. Another dose was given two months later when vomiting began to recur. He quickly returned to normal health with no further relapses. Furthermore, his personality improved and his weight increased beneficially.

"Personality improvement often accompanies successful homeopathic treatment. English homeopath and author Dorothy Shepherd reports returning home to find her puppy lying almost unconscious in its basket. He was pale, barely breathing and drib-bling saliva. Though his nose was warm, the rest of his body was icy cold. Drug treatment probably couldn't have saved him. Dr. Shepherd quickly gave him a homeopathic remedy made from camphor that seemed to match his symptoms.

"In a remarkably short time he opened his eyes, and feebly tried to lick her fingers, which she had dipped in warm milk dosed with a drop or two of brandy. The next morning he crawled out of his basket and was lying by the fire, gaily wagging his tail, when his mistress awoke. Not only was his illness cured, his personality was greatly improved.

"Next comes the case of a four-year old English bulldog with recurrent, unresponsive eruptions between his front toes. Looking like large blue marbles, they would periodically swell, burst and disappear—only to recur again. An allopathic vet had diagnosed the problem as a 'staph' infection and had given antibiotic injections which had had no effect.

"His owners then took him to a local homeopathic vet who gave him Hepar sulph and Ignatia in combination. This stopped the formation of the blue marbles but brought an unpleasant personality change. He became so aggressive that he attacked all sorts of objects, incessantly tortured other dogs, clamped his teeth on his leash and refused to let go, and barked without interruption for as long as eight hours.

"When the case was referred to me, it clearly looked like homeopathic suppression had taken place, i.e. the improper combination remedy, treating only symptoms, had aggravated the overall condition instead of curing it. The original complaint had been replaced by emotional deterioration. Causticum 6x, followed by 10M, brought only slight improvement, so I went on to Tarentula hispanica 200 and then Belladonna 10M. A blue cyst reappeared between the front toes and the dog seemed extremely fatigued and bloated during hot weather.

"Apparently the Belladonna had been close enough to produce a response. The fuller aspect of the disease could now be seen, and I gave Sulphur 10M, which brought marked improvement.

"All the emotional symptoms disappeared and the dog became lovable again. After three months, the excessive barking returned. Another dose of Sulphur 10M produced no improvement, and objectionable behavior increased. Looking at his history and the remaining symptoms, I now prescribed a single dose of Lycopodium 10M. This brought lasting improvement and the owners report that lingering problems are insignificant, with no further relapses. A final remedy may still be required.

"This case illustrates the need to bring the patient back, step by step, from suppression from combination remedies before emotional improvement can finally occur.

"I once treated a cat that had spontaneously undergone a drastic personality change. Where before she had been friendly, now she was irritable, objected to being held and was generally stand-offish. Homeopathic treatment with Nux vomica quickly restored her normal affectionate personality.

"To summarize, when I am able to clearly recognize a patient's unique symptom picture—on the mental, emotional and physical levels—and can match it to the right remedy, I can be certain the patient will respond. Though it's not always easy to make such a match, when I succeed I can count on this principle like I count on gravity."

For fascinating and detailed strategies for taking better care of your household pets, see *Natural Health for Dogs and Cats*, by Richard H. Pitcairn and Susan Pitcairn ($10.95 paper) from most homeopathic suppliers.

Children's Cases

Now let's turn from pets to children ... in cases from the files of Hawaii naturopath Michael Traub.

When Sara was brought in at the age of four with chronic ear problems, her medical history was already extensive. Beginning at the age of two months, she had experienced 48 hours of fever after each of her DPT vaccinations. Her ear infections and allergic rhinitis dated back to the age of fourteen months; so did her chronic sore throat. When she was 18 months old, her father left home and Sara felt abandoned. Her asthmatic bronchitis began six months later. By the time she came to Michael, she had already been treated extensively with antibiotics, especially for recurring strep throat.

Michael took the case and gave her Pulsatilla. He also gave her Pele, Hawaii for her persistent cough. Pele is a new isopathic remedy concocted to deal with the throat-irritating "vog," steadily produced by volcanic dust from Kilauea volcano. Kilauea, at this writing, has been continuously erupting for the past eight years, causing substantial allergic problems.

After seven months Sara was greatly improved. She only wheezed when she ate food she was allergic to, and the episodes were brief—only lasting a few hours. She was five now and doing well in kindergarten, not reacting anymore to dust, cats or mold. Her mother told Michael it was the healthiest she'd ever been in her life. Sara's never had another ear infection.

"Do you see this as a vaccine-related case? " I asked.

"Very possibly. The DPT vaccine could easily have weakened her immune system and predisposed her to getting those recurrent ear and throat infections, asthma and allergies."

Kai Nalu, a 20-month old Hawaiian boy, was brought to Michael for a dry persistent barking cough that had lasted four months. There was no congestion, no history of vaccinations, no recent illnesses. Suspecting the "vog," Michael prescribed Pele, Hawaii 6c, twice a day. Within two months the cough was gone, but when his parents ran out of the remedy it returned. As long as Kai takes the remedy he has no problem from the vog. When the volcano finally stops erupting he'll be all right without it.

Gabriel is a five year old boy with a behavioral problem that came on suddenly. One day he came home from school bragging that he'd been in five fights. He had always liked to be the leader when he played, but now he became more haughty and aggressive. The school suspended him for his sudden violence and his concerned mother brought him to Michael.

"I found out his father had moved out not long before and hadn't called Gabriel recently, and his mother had a boyfriend whom he hated. He'd always been very close to his mother, but now she was away more at work. Like his father he was very jealous and possessive. He was also highly competitive, aggressive and unforgiving ... easily upset and quick to anger. Although he'd always been healthy, now he sometimes vomited in the middle of the night."

Because of the symptoms of competitiveness, jealousy and aggressiveness, etc., Michael prescribed Nux vomica. A month later Gabriel had been accepted back in school and was doing much better. The Nux brought him out of the difficulties created by emotional stress in his home life.

Mirana, a three year old girl, also developed a new set of symptoms with mysterious suddenness. A couple of days after being chilled and catching cold, she was taken to the hospital emergency room because she had turned purple after gagging with a cough. The doctors diagnosed the problem as sinus infection and gave her an antibiotic which failed to help. Instead she got worse, vomiting up to six times every night. Ginger drops slowly cleared up her cough, but a cold soon brought on a relapse. Her parents then brought her to Michael.

"I learned that she was angry, rude and scared when she was sick. And all emotional symptoms made the cough worse. She was intensely irritable and intolerant at night and refused to let anyone help her in any way. She displayed a whooping kind of cough that was loose, wet and rattling although her lungs appeared to be clear. Her face got red and her eyes watered when she coughed, and she brought up a clear liquid. Her coughing was worst late at night."

Michael diagnosed "whooping cough tic," a persistent cough that often follows a case of whooping cough, and prescribed a single dose of Drosera 200c. A week later the cough was gone for good and Mirana was healthy again.

Ten year-old Jason was brought to Michael with a history of severe, recurrent ear infections. The hearing in his left ear was impaired, possibly from repeatedly having tubes inserted. Both his tonsils and adenoids had been removed. A pediatrician had told his mother that surgery would be necessary if the the ear didn't heal. Michael found that a third of the eardrum was missing. He also found a number of warts and canker sores.

"I found Jason emotionally sensitive but otherwise quite healthy," he told me. "I gave him Sulphur and a month later his ear was beginning to heal and the warts were smaller. A month after that the eardrum was nearly healed and a recent plane trip had been painless for him."

Then his mother called to report that he'd come back from the mainland with a bad case of hives. The pediatrician had given him antihistamines which temporarily helped but then aggravated the hives. When Jason arrived in the office a few minutes later, hives covered his body, his face and lips were swollen, he was anxious, trembling, his teeth were chattering, his heart rate was accelerated and he was itching terribly all over.

Michael gave him Apis 30C, put him in a cold shower, then wrapped him in cold wet sheets. When Jason showed improvement, Michael gave him Apis 200c and helped him relax with mild hypnosis for 20 minutes.

"When I unwrapped him," said Michael, "the hives were virtually gone. Then I had a chance to look in his ear. The drum was completely healed. I gave him one more dose of Apis 200c and sent him home. At a checkup a few days later, I found him completely healthy."

Allison, four and a half, suffered with recurrent nosebleeds. They were worse on the left, often lasted for hours, were aggravated by heat, activity or exertion and often occurred during sleep. The family had recently moved from Alaska to settle in the islands. Allison's mother had some experience with acute homeopathic treatment and had given Phosphorus effectively for the nosebleeds.

Michael's diagnosis confirmed Phosphorus, so he gave her a dose of 200c. A few days later she had a healing crisis, with crying and nosebleeds, but it soon went away and she swiftly got better.

Eddie suffered from vaccine poisoning. When he received a DPT shot in his leg at the age of two months, the leg swelled and turned hot and Eddie screamed with pain for eight straight hours! The injection site developed a white patch, and several months later Eddie developed convulsive seizures during which his eyes would roll down, his head would drop forward and he would drool uncontrollably. His head was always sweaty when he slept and he developed other white spots. He seemed a delicate child, with fair skin and refined features.

When he was brought to Michael at the age of eight and a half months, Eddie was having five major seizures and ten small ones every day, and he was taking three kinds of drugs in an attempt to control them. Side effects from the drugs had made his gums swell, adversely affected his balance and attention span, and produced constipation. A CT scan revealed three tumors in his brain. There was a strong history of cancer in the family. His condition is called tuberous sclerosis.

"Based on the head sweats, seizures after vaccination and white spots," said Michael, "I prescribed Silica 200c. A month later the constipation was better, the white spots were the same, the seizures were less intense and fewer, he was eating better, talking more and seemed more alert. He was steadily improving and on his way to a cure.

"Then his parents got to fighting about the effectiveness of homeopathy. The father won out and the treatment was discontinued. Immediately all Eddie's benefits disappeared and his symptoms returned. It was tragic. Here was a severe case of vaccination poisoning that was responding beautifully to a clearly indicated homeopathic remedy. But everything was lost when ignorance and prejudice stopped the treatment."

Peggy Chipkin, my mother's homeopath at Hahnemann Clinic, told me about four-year-old Troy, who was brought in for recurring chronic ear infections and partial loss of hearing. Finding him aggressive, hyperactive, jealous, demanding and angry, Peggy gave him Chamomilla and later Medorrhinum. These remedies cleared up the infections and calmed him somewhat but failed to improve his hearing. And the infections always returned.

It gradually became apparent that Troy's infections always came back following the departure of fond visiting relatives. Troy found these separations hard to accept, weeping and clinging excessively. And gradually this became his normal behavior, replacing the aggressive irritability. At the same time his hearing became worse. Peggy gave him Pulsatilla for his weepy grief and his chronic ear problems.

At the follow-up one month later, Troy's mother reported a fifty percent improvement in his hearing, a great reduction in his weepiness, a new willingness to accept the departure of favorite relatives and a return to normal but less aggressive behavior. "It may take several months," Peggy predicted, "but I expect his ears to fully clear."

Eighteen-month-old Brian was brought to Peggy with bi-lateral pneumonia so severe that she felt she'd be forced to resort to antibiotics for relief (even though they might further weaken him), if she couldn't find the right remedy—fast. Peggy tried Kali Carbonicum for his early morning cough, but it didn't help. Neither did Belladonna for a fever that rose to 103 at midnight and noon. After laboring five days without success, Peggy decided to try one more remedy before reluctantly falling back on antibiotics.

Struggling to decide between Arsenicum and Pulsatilla, she noticed how upset Brian got when his nose dripped on his shirt or his sleeve got caught while putting on his jacket. Despite his age and violent illness, Peggy recognized "fastidiousness," an Arsenicum trait, so that's what she prescribed. After three doses spread over twelve hours, Brian's temperature dropped, his lungs cleared, his cough was nearly gone and he was sleeping peacefully. On a recent checkup, Peggy found him completely healthy.

Books could be filled with similar cases. But this brief sample should show that homeopathy's great effectiveness can't possibly be due to placebo response or healing through belief ... because kids and dogs don't lie!

13

An Embarrassing Admission

**More Dental Problems ... Dr. Deanne Cures My Cold ...
Mom's Constitutional ... Follow-Up on Hawaii ... A
Confession of Lust ... Michael Quinn's Dynamite Remedies**

When we returned from Hawaii to the desert in May, we immediately headed for the dentist. Deanne and Gellie were fine, but my
news was bad ... again. I had *another* cavity that had to be filled
within six months to avoid a root canal. To complicate matters, the
decay was deep under a silver filling and the slow speed drill Dave
had used six months before didn't pack enough power to do the job.

Furthermore, he discovered periodontal disease between two
back molars and urged immediate gum surgery. I groaned. My
dental problems were bigger than ever. It made me wonder if
homeopathy was helping my mouth! But I still wasn't willing to risk
antidoting the Tuberculinum—even though Bill doubted it was
working. What to do?

Dave suggested using an old belt-driven hand drill he used for
making models. It would be slow but there was plenty of torque. I
told him to go ahead. It got so hot he had to stick it under a water
faucet several times a minute to cool it down, but after wearing
out three drill bits the job was done. Then he drilled out the temporary filling in the tooth he'd filled last October—to see if decay
had infected the nerve. It hadn't—another triumph for my vital
force.

The following Friday I had a date with Bill in Berkeley, right after I took my mother to see homeopath Peggy Chipkin, FNP. It had been a long struggle getting Mom to Hahnemann, but finally she'd admitted that her various doctors (the cardiologist, the cancer man, the nose and throat specialist, the chiropractor and the shrink) hadn't helped her much, though the first three gave her increasingly powerful drugs whose side effects sent her reeling.

Last December she'd had the hysterectomy for uterine cancer that Bill recommended. Then her doctor told her she needed five weeks of radiation treatment "to be sure." They didn't tell her, of course, that the radiation damage to her immune system would leave her far more susceptible to illness of all kinds. In close succession she'd had a series of colds, earaches and backaches, with nonstop drainage down the back of her throat. I'd told her she'd enjoy talking to a sympathetic physician about ALL her problems—past and present, physical and emotional. When I promised to pay for her constitutional visit with Peggy, and to take her to the Clinic and hold her hand—she finally agreed to go.

Five days before heading to Berkeley, Deanne and I hiked to the Echo cabin for an overnight visit. That night the temperature dropped to 27 degrees and I managed to get chilled. The next morning I had a nasty cold—only five days before Bill was due to take my case. Cold symptoms can confuse a remedy picture for a homeopath by displacing the chronic symptoms he's seeking. And Deanne hadn't brought along her box of magic remedies.

But left over from the previous summer we found vials of Aconite and Gelsemium. Aconite is a remedy for chill-induced colds. I took it and overnight I was fifty percent better. Gelsemium is also given for colds, so I took that next and got added relief. When we returned to the desert, Dr. Deanne immediately sat down with her books. In half an hour she had matched my symptoms to Allium cepa (raw onion), a remedy she'd never used before. I took it and the miracle happened again. In the morning I was fully recovered ... with three days to spare before journeying to Berkeley!

At the appointed time on Friday I took my mother to Hahnemann and introduced her to Peggy. When the three of us were seated, Peggy asked Mom, "What's bothering you most?" "My throat," Mom replied, sitting ramrod straight.

"How does it bother you?" Peggy coaxed.

"It's so raw I can't sing. And I *love* to sing."

"What do you think makes it raw?"

"Post nasal drip, of course." My usually loquacious mother wasn't giving very much.

Then I remembered I'd urged her not to be verbose. I put my arm around her and turned to Peggy. "Excuse me for interrupting, but since I'm here to help, let me give you a little background. Last winter Mom had a hysterectomy for uterine cancer, followed by five weeks of radiation which weakened her resistance. Since then she's caught every bug that's come along. Now she's here to see if homeopathy can help."

Mom nodded, Peggy smiled and in a minute they were chatting like old friends. I left to do some errands, knowing Hahnemann homeopaths allowed an hour and a half for constitutional interviews. When I returned, I looked for Mom in the waiting room. I should have known better. It was *two* and a half hours before she emerged from Peggy's office. But she was radiant.

"It's the first time a doctor has listened to the *whole* story," she beamed. "It's wonderful to be able to tell someone who understands, someone who can put it all together. And she thinks she can help."

When I asked her what Peggy had prescribed she said, "Nothing, yet. She needs some time to study my case. She'll send around my medicine in a couple of days." I wasn't surprised that Peggy needed time to sort out my mother's eventful eighty-one year history.

When pharmacist Michael Quinn had filled his last prescription he came out to give me the schedule of weekend classes. One long weekend every month the Hahnemann College of Homeopathic Medicine convenes at the Clinic. Its students, all physicians, leave their practices to congregate for instruction in homeopathic theory and detailed symptom pictures of the major remedies. Michael invited me to sit in. By then it was four thirty and time to see Bill.

When I told him I'd replaced my old reading glasses with a new pair at half the magnification, he said, "Good. Use your glasses as little as possible. Your eyes should keep getting better, if you give them some help."

Next I told him about my mysterious breakdown in mid-February: the stone bruises, tendonitis, slit eyelid, wrenched knee and tennis elbow, followed by Ken's flu. "The only symptom that didn't go away was the slit eyelid. Finally I realized that Calendula was making it worse. If I'm allergic to Calendula, what does that leave me?"

"Right," Bill said, deadpan. "If you react to Calendula, you might have to use nothing the rest of your life!" He laughed at my chagrin.

"But we rely on Calendula," I grumbled. "It's ideal for sunburn and a lot of other things."

"Hmmm," he gazed at the ceiling. "Maybe *I* should try it. I go to a ballgame and get a blazing sunburn and then I put on vitamin E. It's crazy that I don't think of Calendula. I think I'll give it a try."

Having found a new, if unlikely, convert for Calendula, I told him about the cold I caught the week before at Echo, and the succession of remedies Deanne had given me—Aconite, Gelsemium and finally Allium cepa. I braced myself for a rebuke, but Bill just nodded.

I had made up my mind to tell him something quite personal, and now I couldn't put it off any longer. "There's something else," I began. "I'd always assumed that my level of . . . uh . . . I guess you'd call it lust . . . was normal in a healthy heterosexual male. But there's been a steady decline." I waited for a reaction.

"Is that good or bad?" His face was expressionless.

"Oh, for me it's good!"

"So it's not . . . a problem? When the circumstance is right you don't have any . . . trouble?"

"Oh, *no!*" I saw he'd misunderstood! "Maybe 'lust' isn't the right word. I'd always assumed that the wandering eye, the urge to pursue and flirt with other women was perfectly normal."

Comprehension lit his face. "So you never understood that that was a mild pathology?"

"No, not until it started to go away! It was a great relief not to have that excess drive anymore."

Bill smiled. "That's a Tuberculinum trait."

"Is it?"

"You didn't know that?"

"No! I'll be darned!"

He chuckled. "Yeah, that's a *great* confirmation. In fact it's classic. I probably should have asked you about that in the beginning. But it's a hard thing to check out. Tuberculinums don't understand the normality. To them the way they are is perfectly natural. But there's a big difference in sex drive between a *driving* need and a freedom."

"I see that—now."

"That was a big problem in sanitoriums in the old days. The only cure for Tuberculosis then was to send patients up to the mountains. But they had a terrible time keeping the sexes apart. These Tuberculinums all wanted to jump in bed with each other." He laughed ... then turned serious. "So, the Tuberculinum's been doing the job the whole time. That's what I believe, now! Pretty amazing!" He shook his head.

"So the next big test will be in the fall when the pollens come out. This year I don't want you taking isopathics. Period! Let's see how far the Tuberculinum takes you. I think you'll continue to get better. But if I were you I'd go easy on acute remedies. They don't seem to have interfered, but you don't want to take a chance screwing up the Tuberculinum. You ought to be sick for a significant amount of time, before you take an acute."

"Really? Why?"

"You need to be sure that acute symptoms have replaced the chronic in your body's priorities. When the body's sick enough, it turns its healing attention from the chronic condition to the current trauma. That's a law of nature and has nothing to do with homeopathy. When that happens, there's not much danger of an acute remedy interfering with a chronic. It's a rule of thumb."

"So, the sicker you are, the safer it is."

"Right. For example, if you feel a cold coming on and you've got a tennis tournament coming up tomorrow and you say to yourself, 'I'm gonna nip this in the bud,' that could be dangerous. If you took the acute but were wrong about the cold, you might interfere with your chronic remedy."

"Okay. If I feel a cold coming I'll take vitamin C."

"Right. Don't take a chance". He put his stack of notes into my folder and closed it. "Okay, I'm not going to prescribe. The Tuberculinum is holding beautifully. It's done so much over such a long period. We have to be extra super careful not to mess with it."

"What do you think brought on my February breakdown?"

"You must have overdone the exercise with all that tennis and basketball and swimming and mountain climbing ... in combination with the emotional stress of your political problems. Plus the return of old symptoms. On top of that you caught a heavy flu from your guest, probably because you were run down. With all that stress, *anybody'd* have a breakdown—I don't care *how* strong their vital force is."

The conversation turned to Michael Quinn's latest succussion machine, the MQ II. Bill was ecstatic. "The remedies he's making us now are *dynamite!* Roger and I noticed the difference simultaneously. We're getting *great* results."

The office door opened and Michael came in.

"We were just talking about you and your fantastic machine, and how you come in the middle of the night to make sure everything's okay. You must be sleep-deprived to a major degree."

Michael permitted himself a small smile. Bill turned back to me. "There's been a quantum leap forward in remedies. At first we planned a double blind study, in which Michael wouldn't tell us which remedies he was giving us, his or Boiron's. We soon dropped it and went with Michael's remedies exclusively. The difference was too great. We didn't want to deprive our patients of the best."

Michael modestly elaborated. "Bill started seeing major aggravations, followed by major improvements. So did Roger. One of Bill's patients, after taking her remedy, had by far the worst migraine headache of her life on Friday, told off her husband on Saturday and by Monday felt better than she had her whole life." He smiled.

Bill nodded. "And she's stayed that way ever since."

After Michael left, Bill said, "He's a wonder. He won't settle for second best. That's why we've got what may be the best remedies in the world. For instance, we want him to make Calcarea from oyster shell, but he won't use mere American oysters. Oh, no! His have to come from the North Sea because that's where Hahnemann got his. He's having oyster shell shipped from somewhere in Scandinavia. He won't be happy until he gets the real thing."

Later that evening in the Pharmacy laboratory, Michael showed me the nook where he makes low potency remedies by hand. "Hahnemann wrote that he'd succuss his remedies by striking his vial of tincture sharply, anywhere from ten to a hundred times, on a book," he explained. "George likes forty, so that's what I use—since it's close to the median. And I use this book." He held up a thick book, smiling faintly.

I chuckled. It was Hahnemann's *Organon*. "So your remedies have all been thumped against the bible?"

He nodded. "It seemed an appropriate choice. Nothing gets changed from the way Hahnemann did it, unless the changes can be proved to be safe improvements. Despite all this caution, I'm trying to establish a new standard of pharmaceutical excellence. So I exhaustively test the innovations I dream up before I introduce them."

He took me into the hospital-white cubicle to see his newest creation, the MQ II. With its shiny stainless steel casing and glittering metallic hoses it looked like a space age robotic octopus. Gone were the Rube Golberg arms and levers of last September. "What happened to the old machine?" I asked.

I thought I saw him wince. "I trashed it. Actually I cannibalized it. We were able to reuse some of the pieces. Even this one is pretty primitive. Biology is 150 years behind physics."

"How much better is this machine?"

"That's total speculation. But I believe it's in every way superior. Of course, results are all that count. You'll have to find out from Bill and Roger and the others. Clinical impressions—though highly subjective—are the only valid test of any medicine."

14

The Case Against Vaccination

Homeopath Richard Moskowitz, MD, Explains Why Routine
Immunization is Dangerous, Ineffective and Often
Unnecessary ... How to Legally Avoid it ... A Guide to
Individual Vaccines

I feel compelled to return to the subject of vaccination because its
threat is so insidious and widespread. Millions of innocent, trusting
Americans unquestioningly rely on a benevolent Uncle Sam to protect them against the spread of communicable disease by means of
the pseudo magic known as vaccination.

When the Dept. of Public Health pundits decree that innoculation is necessary, people everywhere dutifully roll up their sleeves
and submit to injections of some unknown foreign substance that
may well change their lives—and not for the better. And they trust-
ingly turn over their babies and small children for innoculations
that may well afflict their health the rest of their lives. They do so
because they've been led to believe by the doctors, the drug industry and the government that immunization is safe, effective and
necessary.

Unfortunately, it is none of the above!

Homeopaths shudder at the irreparable damage done by vaccination to the nation's health in the name of 'the general welfare.'
As George Vithoulkas points out in *The Science of Homeopathy*,
"vaccination has a profoundly disturbing effect on health, particularly in relation to chronic diseases."

"The Case Against Immunization" was admirably presented several years ago by Richard Moskowitz, MD in the Journal of the American Institute of Homeopathy. My digest of that treatise (mostly in Dr. Moskowitz's words) is here presented to aid understanding and fortify the readers' (especially parents') resolve to refuse to participate in dangerous, unproven, ineffective government programs to immunize. The veteran doctor begins....

"For the past ten years I have felt a deep and growing compunction against routine immunization for children. It began with the fundamental belief that people have the right to make that choice for themselves. Surely the public is entitled to convincing proof that artificial immunization is safe and effective, and that the threat of natural diseases remains sufficiently clear and urgent to warrant mass innoculation of everyone, even against their will if necessary.

"Unfortunately, no such proof has ever been given. The fact remains that they are *compulsory*, that all children are required to undergo them, without sensitive regard for basic differences in individual susceptibility. Furthermore, the attempt to eradicate entire microbial species from the biosphere must inevitably upset the balance of nature in fundamental ways we can as yet scarcely imagine.

"I want to put the case against vaccine immunization as clearly and forcefully as I can, in part, because the growing refusal of parents to vaccinate their children is so seldom articulated ... or taken seriously.

"The customary assumption that the precipitous decline in various natural infections is *attributable* to vaccines remains unproven and continues to be questioned by eminent authorities in the field. Whooping cough, for example, had already begun its steep decline long before the pertussis vaccine was introduced. The same is true for diptheria, tetanus, TB, cholera, typhoid and other common scourges of a bygone era. They all began to disappear toward the end of the nineteeth century, partly in response to improved public health and sanitation—long before antibiotics, vaccines or other medical measures were designed to eradicate them.

"The great microbiologist Rene Dubos observed, 'Men can live peacefully with their most notorious microbial enemies. Millions of young people become infected by polio viruses, yet very few suffer any harm. Infection can occur without producing disease.'"

The whole philosophy of vaccination, it seems clear, reflects the allopathic refusal to consider individual susceptibility!

"The diseases in question have continued to break out even in highly immunized populations. In a recent outbreak of whooping cough, for instance, 46 of the 85 fully immunized children studied contracted the disease.... At UCLA campus in 1977, 34 cases of measles were reported in a population that was supposedly 91% immune.... Although the overall incidence of measles in the U.S. has dropped sharply since the early 1960's, the death rate has remained exactly the same, and the risk of complications such as pneumonia and liver ailments has actually increased.

"These discrepancies could be explained by postulating that vaccines confer only partial or temporary immunity. The vaccine is a 'trick,' i.e. it only *simulates* the natural immune response developed while recovering from the disease. So it is not surprising that artificial immunity will 'wear off' quite easily. There is no way to know how long it will last, because of the many individual variables that would have determined susceptibility to the natural disease."

A number of investigators have shown that, once it wears off, repeated booster doses will have little or no effect. Furthermore, vaccines commonly produce a variety of symptoms of their own ... in some cases considerably more serious than the original disease, involving deeper or more vital organs. These symptoms are also often difficult to recognize and fail to disappear spontaneously.

"In a recent outbreak of mumps in supposedly immune children, several developed atypical symptoms such as anorexia, vomiting and rashes. Atypical measles can be much more severe than the regular kind, with pneumonia, petechiae, edema and severe pain. Evidence such as this makes it less and less plausible to assume that vaccines produce a good likeness of true or healthy immunity.

"I will present a few of my own vaccine cases, partly to ask the crucial question: how do vaccines actually *work?* In my first case, an 8-month old girl exhibited recurrent episodes of fever of unknown origin. The mother said that all episodes were exactly one month apart and that the first one started one month after her last DPT injection. Moreover, the child had had similar episodes at the time of her other injections, but the pediatrician had dismissed them as 'common' reactions to the vaccine!

"The DPT connection was confirmed by giving the diluted homeopathic vaccine orally, followed by complete recovery, with no more episodes of any kind.

"Since then I have seen many other cases of children with recurrent fevers of unknown origin which were similarly traceable to the pertussis vaccine, and which responded successfully to the homeopathic DPT vaccine. I believe the pertussis vaccine to be one of the major causes of recurrent fevers of unknown origin in small children today.

"In another case, personally known but not treated by me, a 5-year old boy came down with chronic lymphocytic leukemia following a DPT vaccination. He was twice treated successfully with homeopathic remedies, with spleen and liver shrinkage to nearly normal size, but followed by full relapse soon after each DPT booster.

"It is dangerously misleading and, indeed the exact opposite of the truth to claim that a vaccine makes us 'immune' or *protects* us against an acute disease, if it only drives the disease deeper into the interior and causes us to harbor it *chronically*, such that our responses to it become progressively weaker, and show less and less tendency to heal or resolve themselves spontaneously.

"There is substantial evidence that the maturation of the immune system is actually stimulated by developing and recovering from such childhood diseases as measles. The "illness" that we know as measles is precisely the definitive effort of the immune system to clear the virus from the blood.

"The process of *mounting* an acute illness like measles, no less than recovering from it, involves a general mobilization of the entire immune system. Such illnesses are decisive experiences in the normal maturation of the immune system as a whole. The child who recovers from measles will never again be susceptible to it.

The ability to mount a vigorous acute response of this type must therefore be reckoned among the most fundamental requirements of general health and well-being.

"In contrast, when an artificially attenuated virus such as measles is injected directly into the blood, bypassing the normal portal of entry, there is no generalized inflammatory response, no incubation period of local contact, and very little possibility of eliminating the virus via the same route. By 'tricking' the body in this fashion, we have accomplished something that the entire immune system seems to have evolved to prevent: we have placed the virus directly into the blood, and given it free and immediate access to the major immune organs and tissues, without any obvious way of getting rid of it.

"The result is, indeed, the production of circulating antibodies, but the price that we have to pay for them is the persistence of the virus in the blood for prolonged periods, perhaps permanently, which in turn presupposes a systematic weakening of our ability to mount an effective response to other acute infections as well. Artificial immunization focuses on *antibody production,* a single aspect of the immune process.

"Far from producing a genuine immunity, these vaccines may actually interfere with or *suppress* the immune response as a whole. By making it difficult to mount a vigorous acute response to infection, artificial immunizations tend to substitute a much weaker *chronic* response, with little or no tendency to heal itself spontaneously.

"Adequate models already exist for predicting what sorts of chronic disease are likely to result from the chronic, long-term persistence of viruses and other foreign proteins within the cells of the immune system. 'Latent viruses' have already been implicated in three distinct types of chronic disease: (1) *recurrent or episodic acute diseases* such as herpes, shingles, warts, etc., (2) *'slow virus' diseases,* and (3) *tumors*, both benign and malignant.

"The latent virus survives as a clearly 'foreign' element within the cell, which means the immune system must continue to make antibodies to protect against it. The persistence of live viruses cannot fail to provoke *auto-immune* phenomena, in which the body attacks and attempts to destroy its own tissues. Since routine vaccination introduces live viruses into the blood of vast numbers of people, it is difficult to escape the conclusion that a significant harvest of auto-immune diseases must automatically result.

"Latent viruses, auto-immune phenomena and cancer seem to represent different aspects of the same basic dilemma, which the immune system can neither escape nor resolve. All of them presuppose a certain degree of *chronic immune failure*, a state in which it becomes difficult or impossible for the body either to recognize it's own cells as unambiguously its own, or to eliminate its parasites as unequivocably foreign. Since this precarious balance may break down at any time, latent viruses are like biological 'time bombs,' set to explode at an indeterminate time in the future.

"Auto-immune diseases have always seemed obscure, aberrant and bizarre, because it is not obvious why the body should suddenly begin to attack and destroy its own tissues. They make a lot more sense, and indeed must be reckoned as 'healthy,' if destroying chronically infected cells is the only possible way of eliminating an even more serious threat to life, namely, the persistence of the foreign antigens within the cells of the host.

"If what I am saying turns out to be true, the attempt at artificial immunization has caused us to trade the acute epidemic diseases of the past century for the far less curable chronic diseases of the present. In doing so, we have opened up the limitless evolutionary danger of *in vivo* genetic recombination within the cells of the race.

"I want next to consider the vaccines on an individual basis.

"MMR is composed of attenuated live measles, mumps and rubella (German measles) viruses administered in a single injection. Prior to the vaccine era, measles, mumps and rubella were reckoned among the 'routine childhood diseases.' Yet measles can be devastating when a population encounters it for the first time. The evolution of a disease like measles from dreaded killer to an ordinary disease of childhood presupposes the development of nonspecific or 'herd' immunity in young children, such that when they are finally exposed to the disease, it activates defense mechanisms already prepared and in place.

"The death rate from measles is very low, the incidence of

serious complication insignificant, and the general benefit to the child who recovers is very great. It therefore seems unreasonable to vaccinate children against measles, especially considering the high probability of auto-immune diseases, cancer, and whatever else may result from the propagation of latent measles virus in human tissue culture for life.

"The case for immunizing against mumps and rubella seems even more tenuous. Like measles, mumps is fast becoming a disease of adolescents and young adults, which age groups tolerate it much less well. The greatest favor we could do for our children would be to expose them to measles and mumps when they are young, which would protect them against contracting the more serious forms of these diseases when they are older, and greatly assist in their immunological maturation with minimal risk."

The same is true of rubella, which in young children is so mild that it frequently escapes detection. The vaccine was developed to prevent CRS, congenital rubella syndrome. But here again, the simplest and most effective way to prevent CRS would be to expose everybody to rubella in elementary school. Re-infection does sometimes occur, but (ironically) much less often than after vaccination against rubella!

"Diphtheria and tetanus are still serious, sometimes fatal diseases." This is especially true of tetanus, which carries a mortality rate of close to fifty percent. Diphtheria and tetanus vaccines are made from certain toxins produced by them, not from the living organisms themselves. These 'toxoids' therefore do not protect against infection *per se*, but only against the systemic effect of the corresponding poisons. "Moreover, both diseases are readily controlled by simple sanitary measures and careful attention to wound hygiene. And both have been steadily disappearing from the developing countries since long before the vaccines were introduced."

Diphtheria now occurs only sporadically in the United States. When it does break out, fully immunized children are almost as likely to contract the disease as those who have not been vaccinated! So diptheria toxoid seems not to have produced a genuine immunity to diphtheria at all, but rather some sort of chronic immune *tolerance* ...with long-term suppressive effects on the immune system generally. All the DPT vaccines are also prepared with potentially toxic chemical preservatives, so that the antigenic challenge will continue for as long as possible.

"Tetanus toxoid likewise presumably survives for years or even decades as a potent foreign antigen, with long-term effects on the immune system and elsewhere that cannot at present be measured.

"Whooping cough, like diphtheria and tetanus, began to decline as a serious threat long before the pertussis vaccine was introduced. Moreoever, the vaccine has not been particularly effective, and the incidence of known side-effects is disturbingly high.

"Pertussis vaccine has become controversial even in the U.S., where medical opinion has remained almost unanimous in favor of immunization generally. The power of pertussis vaccine to damage the central nervous system is well known. Pressure to immunize against whooping cough at present seems attributable to the higher death rate of the disease in very young infants, which has led to the terrifying practice of giving this most dangerous of vaccines to infants two months of age, in spite of the fact that their mothers' milk would normally have protected them from *all* infections about as well as can be done.

"For all of these reasons, routine pertussis immunization should be discontinued as quickly as possible, and more studies should be made to assess and compensate the damage that has already been done.

"Poliomyelitis and the polio vaccines are entirely different.... The poliovirus produces no symptoms whatsoever in over ninety percent of the people who contract it, even under epidemic conditions. And only 1-2 percent of those who do become chronically ill ever progress to full-blown 'poliomyelitis,' with its characteristic and devastating neurological picture. This disease presupposes a specific *anatomical* susceptibility in certain individuals, while in the population at large, natural immunity to poliovirus by the 1950's was already as close to being universal as it can ever be.

"Perhaps we should not attempt to beat nature at her own game: to eliminate a problem that cannot be eliminated, i e. the susceptibility to disease itself. I am deeply troubled by the atmosphere of fanaticism with which vaccines are imposed on the public, while serious discussion of them is ignored or stifled by the medical authorities."

Not until 1978 did congress charge the American Academy of Pediatrics with responsibility to formulate guidelines for Federal compensation for "vaccination-related" injuries. Unfortunately, the resulting eligibility restrictions excluded all conditions arising more than 30 days following immunization! That excludes all chronic diseases and all conditions not previously recognized as vaccine-related, (i.e. all *new* information on vaccine injuries)!

"Neither the government nor the medical establishment can be ignorant of the possibility lurking in every parent's heart that vaccines cause cancer and other chronic diseases.

"As Rene Dubos points out, 'The faith in the magical power of drugs ... comes close at times to mass hysteria.' We prefer to forget the older and simpler truth that susceptibility to illness is deeply rooted in our own biological nature, and that the phenomena of disease are simply the expression of our own life energy, trying to overcome whatever it is trying to overcome, trying in short to *heal* itself. We are all genuinely at risk of illness and death at every moment, and no amount of technology can change that.

"The miracle of life has given us illness and disease, but it has also given us the arts of medicine and healing, and sometimes an awareness of health and well-being that transcends all boundaries. That is *my* religion, and while I willingly share it, I would not *force* it on anybody."

Bill Gray agrees with Dr. Moskowitz. "His accusations about the cavalier arrogance of the allopaths is 'right on,' and his political complaints are unassailable. Vaccines are potent foreign substances usually administered by a route different from that of the natural infection. This bypasses hosts of natural immune mechanisms essential to conferring complete immunity."

Having now been warned successively by such experienced authorities as George Vithoulkas, Richard Moskowitz and Bill Gray, I hope the reader—especially new parents—will think twice before submitting themselves or their children to routine allopathic vaccination.

And don't be intimidated by school officials who threaten, "No shots, no school!"

There is no such thing as compulsory vaccination!! And there are no federal vaccination laws. But don't expect public officials to admit it. Every state in the union has exemptions to its laws for "medical" or "religious" reasons. And you don't have to be a member of a church to refuse on religious or philosophical grounds. A private belief or conviction is sufficient. These loopholes were built-in to protect the government from liability, not to protect the public from being poisoned, but they work both ways.

If you check the exemptions in the law at your local library, deal with officials firmly and in writing, you are absolutely sure to prevail. The exemptions also apply to world travelers and people in military service. If you don't want vaccinations for yourself or your children, no one can force you to take them, nor can you be denied rights and privileges because you refuse. But many bureaucrats will make it seem otherwise.

Dr. Moskowitz strongly urges avoidance of vaccination by anyone with a strong family history of vaccine reaction or with blood relatives who have suffered from severe or complicated cases of any of the diseases mentioned here. These people have a much greater risk of adverse reactions. Other good grounds for medical exemptions from vaccination include preexisting epilepsy, central nervous system disorder, certain allergies, constitutional weakness, any severe or disabling chronic disease ... or even temporary poor health.

Most homeopaths believe that children are better off acquiring immunity from these now rare and generally mild diseases by actually contracting the diseases themselves while young. Hahnemann Clinic keeps a list of kid-patients who have not yet had measles. When one of them contracts it, arrangements are made to have the child play for a few hours with the others, in order to induce the disease!

A woman who contracts Rubella in her first three months of pregnancy risks serious damage to her baby. So a woman of child-bearing age who has not had Rubella should therefore be allopathically immunized to protect her baby during pregnancy.

The only immunizations Bill Gray recommends to his patients are polio and tetanus. "But I want people to think the matter through, weigh the risks and the benefits and make their own decisons. Tetanus vaccine, since world War II, has seemed very safe—perhaps because the disease is caused by puncture wounds and the vaccine is similarily injected. Of course the best prevention of disease of all kinds is homeopathic constitutional treatment. Though sometimes slow and difficult, it's safe, effective and inexpensive."

Parents still agonizing over what to do for their babies might well read further. I highly recommend *DPT, A Shot in the Dark*, co-authored by Harris L. Coulter, and *Homeopathy in Epidemic Diseases* by Dorothy Shepherd.

Knowledge brings the power to protect your children from disease itself and from the sometimes hidden risks of vaccination.

15

Second Summer Adventures

At Homeopathic Medical School ... A Test of Stamina ...
Gum Surgery ... Building First Aid Kits ... Taking Stock of
Gains ... Mom's Benefits ... A Dozen Cured Cases
by Dr. Deanne

At nine o'clock on a fine May morning I stepped into the jam-packed Clinic library. Twenty students of all descriptions were wedged into a variety of chairs at four rows of tables. I watched them scribbling in big notebooks, muttering as they consulted thick reference books, occasionally chuckling, but always intent on the lecturer standing at the head of the class. All they seemed to have in common was their enthusiasm for homeopathy and the unpretentiousness of their dress. This was Hahnemann College of Homeopathic Medicine in action.

The lecturer was Jonathan Shore, MD. He spoke with a soft English accent about the vital force as perceived by James Tyler Kent, elaborating on the philosophical foundations of homeopathy. "The least important symptoms are those that are coarse and common," Jonathan told us, "while the fine or subtle symptoms are always most revealing. Disease may be defined as a change of state." And "true disease is totally systemic, permeating the entire organism."

All I knew about the students around me was that each was a professional physican who had paid $6,000 for the priviledge of leaving his or her family and practice one 4-day weekend every month for two years, to come tens or hundreds of miles to study under some of the best classical homeopaths in America. They seemed caring people first and physicans second. Their yearning to heal seemed to give the room warmth.

"Everything a patient says is fascinating to a homeopath," Jonathan was saying, "and that deep interest stimulates the patient's trust and helps make the system work. It's what allows us to do our jobs effectively." And, "We have no idea—none whatso-ever—what goes on inside the human body." I found this candor refreshing.

Around the middle of the morning Dr. Shore announced a five minute break. Before anyone could move, Michael stood up and introduced me. Beaming faces nodded in my direction, making me feel welcome, and I chatted with my neighbors until the lecture resumed. A few minutes later, Michael raised his hand to ask. "Are there other causes of disease than bacteria?"

"I've changed my views various times on that question," said Jonathan. "Bacteria are everywhere. It can even be postulated that disease arises because we are fixed in our thinking, our beliefs. The real study of a sick man may well be a meditation on his symptoms. We know a man's mind can infect others. Antibiotics, by killing bacteria, merely interrupt a changed state, they don't cure it. Viral illness is nearly always systemic."

A few minutes before noon, Jonathan frowned at his watch and said, "I'm afraid I'm running late. Shall we forget the rest and eat, or shall I go on another fifteen minutes?" "Go on!" was the immedi-ate and unanimous response, despite the fact that everyone had been sitting in hard chairs in a stuffy cramped room for three hours.

It was nearly twelve-thirty when the class broke for lunch. After briefly stretching, most students returned to the library to open bag lunches and talk about homeopathy and their patients, joking and laughing. I hadn't brought anything to eat but the Clinic had provided platters of crackers, cheese and fresh fruit. One stu-dent offered me a bag of pistachio nuts, while another gave me a box of raisins.

Here were chiropractors, MD's, lay prescribers, family nurse practitioners and osteopaths all eating happily together, sharing their food, case histories and experience in homeopathy. Michael and I, still hungry, left to visit a taco stand down the street. By the time we returned, enchiladas in hand, the room was full and buzzing, waiting for the afternoon session to begin. Nancy Herrick, PA, was to present the lecture, a three hour discourse on the remedy picture of Nux vomica.

I hadn't the slightest interest in Nux vomica, but the picture she painted was so enthralling that I found myself taking notes as furiously as the students around me. Michael, now sitting beside me, leaned over to whisper, "Nancy's the best kept secret in the Clinic. She's terrific! I'd put her on a par with Bill and Roger."

"Nux vomica, the poison nut, is largely strichnine," Nancy told us. "The poisons comprise some of our most powerful remedies. Nux is the so-called 'American' remedy because it's picture is so close to what we call the "Type A" personality. Nux is extremely angry and irritable, a workaholic and often an *al*coholic." After delineating the remedy's general characteristics, she proceeded to the physical, mental and emotional characteristics in greater detail—first for infants and children, then adolescents and finally adults, continuing with the progression of the pathology to its final full-blown stages, culminating, in extreme cases, in death.

I remembered the dramatic cure Deanne had produced with Nux on our young friend Danny the summer before at Echo. Listening to a professional present a symptom picture was like listening to the reading of an enthralling story. There was the same buildup of character and suspense. I sat happily to the end, unconscious of the passage of time. The next day was Sunday and I had family commitments, but I found myself wishing I were back in the crowded library with that jolly bunch of budding homeopaths, listening to the unfolding remedy pictures of Ignatia and Natrum muriaticum. And Bill was due to lecture on Monday. It would have been fun to be there and listen.

I had mentioned my attraction to the group to Michael the day before. "I know," he'd nodded. "I like being there, too. When the course is in session I spend all the time there I can. You're welcome to come back anytime."

On Sunday afternoon we drove back over the mountains to the desert. A few days later I learned by phone from my mother that Peggy had given her Natrum muriaticum. It made me wish all the more that I'd heard the remedy presented.

June had come and we'd soon be moving to the cabin for the summer, but first I wanted to take Deanne up nearby Mt. Patterson. It was ten years since I'd climbed it, so the 2,600 foot climb would measure my change in stamina. I found the going easier than I remembered, and after three hours of hard climbing in the chill thin air we stood on top, two vertical miles above the sea. Seven hours and twelve miles after starting, we made it back to the car and headed home. I felt less fatigued and happier than I had ten years earlier, thanks to the rejuvenating work of the Tuberculinum. Not only had it arrested my aging process, it seemed to have turned back the clock!

Shortly after we moved to Echo, I went to the periodontist for gum surgery. Dr. Deanne made sure I was prepared. Moments before surgery she gave me a dose of Arnica 200 for shock and pain. And bulging my pocket was an eye-dropper bottle of Calendula tincture and a small empty bottle. "When they're done," she instructed, "don't let them give you any drugs. Just ask for hot water for your bottle, then put in ten drops of Calendula. Shake it up and swish it around in your mouth. It'll stop any bleeding and start your gums healing immediately."

An hour and a half later when the job was done, the dentist urged me to avoid spicy foods. "You're going to have some pain when the anesthetic wears off," he warned. "And don't be upset if your gums are still bleeding tomorrow." I thanked him and we left for The China Kitchen, a Szechuan restaurant that specializes in hot spicy food. Deanne gave me another dose of Arnica just before we went in. As always, the Kung Pau chicken was smoking and delicious. Before lunch was over the anesthetic wore off, but I had almost no pain, and no bleeding at all.

Late that afternoon my mouth began to ache, but the pain disappeared when Deanne gave me a third dose of Arnica. The next day I felt fine and that night I was able to brush my freshly cut, stitched-up gums without difficulty. Two days later I called the dentist and asked to have the troublesome stitches removed, but he insisted I wait a full week like everybody else. When he saw me he was impressed by the speed with which I'd healed. But I don't think he quite believed that I'd been free of both pain and bleeding from the start.

Deanne had been doing a lot of reading about acute prescribing, and one of her first projects when we moved to the cabin was to ruthlessly clean out our old medicine cabinet. So, into the garbage pail went Tetracycline, Ambesol, Bactine, Rolaids, Tums, Bufferin, Excedrin, Ben Gay, Tylenol, Vicks, Neo-synepherine, Fizrin, Blistex and various other familiar medications. Could homeopathy really improve on all these household staples? I asked. Deanne assured me it could—with greater efficacy, no side effects, and at a fraction of the cost.

"I've made a list of what we need to fill out our kit," she told me, "and I'm calling Michael Quinn today to order." At the moment our kit contained fifty different vials plus Calendula and Hypericum tinctures (liquid), Arnicated oil and Calendula lotion and cerate (salve). She was ordering Ledum tincture for puncture wounds, insect bites and stings; Urtica urens tincture for first degree burns, hives and rashes; Cantharis tincture for third degree burns; Vipera for nose bleeds; Iris for migraine headaches; Glonine for heat induced headaches; Causticum for second degree burns; Graphites for constipation, dermatitis, impetigo, ringworm, yeast infection, vaginitis and styes; Aloe for bowel problems; Tarentula for boils and carbuncles; and Opium for altitude sickness.

She'd been reading a book by Dorothy Shepherd (*Homeopathy for the First Aider*) and she wanted the capability to treat all these maladies. She came back from her canoe trip across the lake to the phone to report that Michael was sending everything except the Opium, which was forbidden. "He told me Cocaine was also good for altitude sickness, but he couldn't sell me that either," she grumped. I wondered why she cared about altitude sickness, since neither of us had ever had it. Perhaps she had a premonition.

Late in June the lodgepole pine forest that surrounded the cabin began to shed it's yellow pollen. Some people were allergic to it, but in twenty-six years I'd never been bothered. This year's crop was gigantic. Old-timers said they hadn't seen so much pollen in sixty years! Our cove was a sheet of rippling gold. A yellow mist filled the basin and every tree and rock was filmed with heavy yellow dust. To my surprise, spots on my face that always itched in the fall now began to trouble me. Calendula helped but they didn't go away. At times the pollen cloud was so thick it almost obscured the lake's far shore. We ate, breathed and slept in pollen.

To get away from it we hastily planned a four-day backpacking trip into the Toiyabe Range in the Nevada desert. Before we left, Deanne examined my ancient backpacking first aid kit with disdain, threw out the old medicines and replaced them with homeopathic remedies.

In a 35 mm plastic film canister she tucked two tiny screw-topped vials of Arnica 200 (for shock, pain, bruises) and Ruta 6 (for sprains or pulled muscles) and packed them with cottonballs (to be used as applicators for lotion and tincture). In a fliptop vial she poured a thimbleful of Hypericum tincture (for cuts and insect bites). Completing the kit was a small squeeze bottle of Calendula lotion, a first aid kit all by itself.

Two days later we were camped in the highest timber more than two miles above the sea in mountains surrounded by desert. It was lunchtime and I was ravenous but Deanne didn't feel hungry. Unfortunately she ate anyway. An hour later she was overcome with violent nausea and stomach cramps. The symptoms were like food poisoning or stomach flu, but we couldn't figure out a likely source of either.

The next day we had planned to climb Arc Dome, the highest peak in the Range. Deanne felt better but was still afraid to eat. She wanted to try for the summit, but if she collapsed or fell and got hurt, there was no way I could carry her out. We hadn't seen another human, and it was forty miles to the nearest help. I was sitting on top when I realized Deanne had altitude sickness! When I returned to explain, she ate everything in sight before we headed back to camp to start home. On the drive back to Echo she told me she'd decided to augment our kit with Arnicated oil and Rhus tox—as well as Urtica urens for the patch of nettles that had stung our legs on the homeward hike.

By now the sores on my face were almost healed. At the cabin we found the pollen storm fading. Yellow dust still coated everything, but the golden haze was gone. When lingering sores on my face began to itch, I treated them with Calendula—until I realized it was making them worse. When I quit they immediately healed. I was reminded of Bill's joke at my expense a month earlier, "Maybe the rest of your life you'll have to use—nothing!"

It was easy for him to say, but I was anxious about the coming onslaught of rabbit brush and sage. If pine pollen, which had never bothered me before, now made me break out, what would the deadly desert pollens do? And if my body refused to tolerate Calendula—and the isopathic remedies were forbidden—how was I supposed to fight back? The only comfort I could find was that this year Bill expected considerable improvement. I'd find out in less than two months!

In the meantime, I was happy, strong and fit. My irritation level continued to decline, and I no longer felt tempted by the maidens in bikinis who smiled at me from passing canoes. I hardly used my weak eyeglasses, except to read by lamplight, and once again I could tie tiny trout flies to my gossamer leader while fishing the lakeshore at dusk. I hadn't been able to do that for a decade!

And I realized I no longer made endless lists—even lists of lists—of things I had to do. I got just as much done in a more relaxed, less ordered manner. Clearly there'd been a subtle shift in my priorities. I wasn't straining as hard to accomplish, and relations of every sort were happier and less stressful. If I was easily irritated it often meant that my nose was blocked, forcing me to breath through my mouth. But that happened less and less. My nose was very slowly getting better.

One morning I awoke suddenly and found myself observing my body as though I were outside it. My nose was partially congested but my body was struggling valiantly to force air through it, keeping my mouth shut. For a lifelong mouth breather it was a revelation. Clearly my body considered mouth breathing an affliction to be overcome. Hopefully that meant I would someday be able to breathe normally all the time ... my lifelong dream!

Down at the Echo marina one afternoon, our novelist friend Lynne complained of a tennis elbow so acutely painful that she couldn't type or sleep. Gingerly she removed her right arm from the sweater pocket she was using as a sling. "I can't touch two fingers together without pain." She demonstrated, wincing. "And I don't even know how to play tennis!" She said she'd been to a doctor who gave her a quart bottle of Motrin in the highest strength made. She'd taken them faithfully for ten straight weeks—without the slightest improvement—but there'd been plenty of side effects. Her feet had swollen until she couldn't put on sandals, and she'd suffered frequent headaches and depression.

"And the doctor said he wouldn't even *talk* to me until I'd finished the whole bottle. When I quit taking the damm things last week in disgust, I immediately lost five pounds of water from my feet!"

"Deanne can help you," I assured her. "She cured my tennis elbow—and tendonitis—last winter." I invited her to come to the cabin the next day. We were barely out of bed when Lynne arrived. After asking a few questions, Deanne gave her Ruta 6, with orders to take it every four hours for 24 hours. We met her the next day at a party and she was beaming. "Look at that," she said, lifting her arm. "Yesterday I couldn't do that. "It's magic! I can't believe it!"

The next morning she paddled her canoe to our pier, beaming. "Look at that!" she said, lifting the paddle with her bad arm and waving it in the air. "It gets better every hour. It's spooky! Tell me all about this homeopathy stuff." Deanne gave her a dose of Ruta 200—and our loaner copy of Vithoulkas' *New Man....* Three months later, a final dose of Ruta 200 cleared up the last of Lynne's symptoms.

A letter from my mother reported that she'd been to see Peggy for a followup. Her congestion and drainage were both much improved and she could sing again. She was delighted.

One day at Echo we were sitting on a dock, watching a swimming race, when one of the contestants, a friend of ours named

Cindy, veered out of her lane and headed straight toward the blade-like prow of an aluminum canoe. Helplessly we watched with horror as she hit with a thud and sank!

Fortunately the water was only waist deep and she staggered to her feet, blood streaming from underneath her nose. She was taken to a doctor, returning sometime later with a bloody butterfly bandage above her lip. Several hours later we met Cindy at dinner. She was still in pain so Deanne gave her Arnica 200. When we saw her again, several weeks later, she thanked Deanne, "for that wonderful stuff you gave me. I had no more pain or swelling after that, and my mouth healed up really fast."

When I talked to my mother a few days later, she asked, "Do you get these sudden feelings of ... well-being?" I told her I felt that way most of the time and urged her to explain. It soon became clear that *her* normal state was mild depression. "These brief periods of well-being—it's almost euphoria. They're just ... marvelous, really wonderful—even if they are rather few and far between." She told me she'd come to like and trust Peggy. Mom's initial reluctance and anxiety about homeopathy seemed to have disappeared.

One August evening we met at a friend's cabin for a bridge game, but Pat was unable to sit down to the table. She had aggravated an old injury to her tailbone, obliging her to stand or lean against a stool. At Deanne's invitation, Pat came to our cabin the next day for a dose of Hypericum 30. As usual, Deanne wrapped enough pellets in a paper packet to last two days, and she dispensed strict instructions regarding coffee, camphor, etc.

The next day Deanne and I were hiking when I was stung by a wasp on my right index finger. The sudden pain was intense. As a boy I'd been so allergic to bee stings that I had to be taken to the doctor, so I expected considerable swelling and pain ... just what I needed on the eve of a river trip in which I'd be rowing more than seventy miles of whitewater!

I jumped up and down, howling with pain, while Deanne opened her pack, got out her tiny homeopathic first aid kit and deftly put a drop of brown Hypericum tincture on the white and widening welt on my finger. Within a single second the pain dropped by fifty percent! Five minutes later I couldn't remember which finger had been stung! And Deanne assured me that Hypericum was only the third best remedy for bee stings. Apis came first, followed by Ledum.

On our return to Echo, we stopped at Pat's cabin. She was jubilant about the improvement Deanne's oral Hypericum had made in her tailbone. For the first time since the injury she'd been able to sleep. She could even sit down, so of course she wanted to play cards. She insisted we stay for supper, which swiftly revived us, and an hour later we were happily playing bridge. Here were two very different Hypericum cures in the space of twenty-four hours.

Six months later Pat called us on a visit to Hawaii to report that she was playing golf and skiing once again with abandon. "And I tell everyone I meet about Deanne and homeopathy and how they put me back in circulation."

The next day, we left for Whitebird, Idaho, and a six day raft trip on the Lower Salmon River. The outfitters, Chuck and Judy Nichols, assured the seventeen of us that while conventional first aid supplies would be on board, "You may want to take your problems to Deanne Wood, who has very effective homeopathic remedies." It turned out that Cindy, the lady who'd split her lip on the canoe, had told Judy about the accident and Deanne's magic Arnica.

We hadn't been on the river two hours before Deanne got her first call for help. She was paddling in the lead boat while I lazily stroked my oar boat and chatted with Ricardo, the Mexican captain of the supply boat. All of a sudden Ricardo slapped his neck, let out a yell and bent his oars, powering past me down the river. He had been stung on the back of the neck by a hornet, and he was highly allergic to bee stings. It was his ninth sting of the season and he groaned that he was in for four days of constant pain and swelling. Deanne put a single drop of Ledum on the red-bordered, white welt the size of a silver dollar on Ricardo's neck.

A look of amazement came over his face. "She stop hurting! She mucho better," he said in awe. "Solamente media!" Half the pain was gone in a matter of seconds. When we beached on a sand-bar to make camp for the night, Ricardo came straight to Deanne. He was beaming as he lifted his long black hair to show her his neck. "That stuff, she *magnifico!*" he told her. "Look! no more bump!"

It was true. The white swollen welt had disappeared. Ricardo's bronze neck now looked perfectly normal. The Ledum had accomplished in less than two hours what usually took four painful days! Our river companions were quietly impressed. Before long they began to sidle up to Deanne to tell her about their problems, wondering what she and her magic kit could do for them.

After a volleyball game on the beach, Thom brought her a painfully abraded hip he had incurred while diving for the ball. Calendula brought immediate relief, just as it did for Karen's sunburn. The next day Deanne gave 13-year-old Teddy Rhus tox for the swelling and eruption of poison oak on his forearms. When she checked him at our lunch stop, the pimples, itching and swelling had disappeared.

Teddy's dad, Lew, complained of pain and swelling in his back brought on by sitting in a cramped raft and paddling hard all morning. Just a month before he'd had spinal surgery to fuse two disks. Now he wondered if he'd made a mistake in coming on a wilderness raft trip so soon. Deanne got out her kit and gave him Arnica. After four doses in twenty-four hours, the pain was greatly reduced. So she switched to Rhus tox for strain. The relief it provided kept him paddling the rest of the trip.

Pleased with the swift relief Calendula had brought to her sunburned shoulders, Karen returned for more for the red abrasions on her legs produced by constant rubbing on the hull of the raft as she paddled.

Captain Judy brought Deanne a painfully swollen finger that had bothered her for weeks, ever since a hangnail had gotten infected. It throbbed with pain when Judy tightly gripped her paddle, which she did for five hours every day. Together, she and Deanne opened the finger, then Deanne treated it with Hypericum four times a day. By the end of the trip Judy's finger was much improved. Like Lew, she'd been able to keep paddling. She vowed she was someday going to Hahnemann for a 'constitutional.' Lots of our friends have.

Before the trip was over, half the crew of seventeen had come to Deanne for homeopathic help ... and that included us. When Deanne happened to bite open the inside of her cheek, she healed it quickly with Calendula. When I lost control of my boat in a big rapid and was catapulted from my seat, she treated my barked shin with Arnicated oil. An hour later the bruise was forgotten.

Back at Echo, September had now arrived and it was time for the ladies to depart for school. I was alone once again, but I didn't really mind. The weather was fine and I had plenty to do. I wasn't in any hurry to descend to the desert to test the Tuberculinum. This year I was supposed to be fifty percent improved. Another two weeks and I'd find out.

16

What Can Homeopathy Cure?

Cancer ... AIDS ... Heart Disease ... Hypertension ...
Arthritis ... Parkinson's ... Multiple Sclerosis ... ALS ...
Arteriosclerosis ... Diabetes ... Child & Female Ailments ...
Injuries ... Epidemics ... Colds & Flus ...
TV Medicines Debunked ... Dentistry ... Insanity

What hope can homeopathy hold out to sufferers of the major afflictions of our time? It would take a shelf of books to fully answer that question. I asked Bill for a quick prognosis so readers could assess the exciting chances of curing the varied ailments of their family and friends.

Conventional medicine, we know, has few if any answers— much less cures. It offers only temporary relief of symptoms or mechanical solutions (like heart bypasses) that ignore the past (i.e. causes) and the future (side effects and relapses). And its expensive treatments often seriously undermine health.

Here's Bill's brief synopsis of what patients can expect from homeopathy.

Cancer

"Broadly speaking, homeopathy can cure cancer. If it's in an early stage and hasn't yet attacked vital organs, cancer is as curable as any other disease. Our cure rate of early stage cancer runs around eighty percent. If it's later stage, that drops to forty or fifty percent.

If the cancer becomes metastisized and the body becomes riddled, then it's more difficult. We can't cure many of those cases."

"Does cancer require constitutional treatment?"

"Right. And the more advanced the case, the more skill and experience are required. Homeopathy has a lot to offer terminal cases, too. We can make the patient better, we can prolong life, and most of all we can palliate (relieve) suffering without clouding the patient's mind with dope."

"What about helping people who've already been treated by surgery, radiation or chemotherapy? Like my mother."

"Homeopathy can help a lot. By treating the patient constitutionally, we can build up health and resistance. So, in essence, we've got help for three different classes of cancer patients. We can cure early stage or light cases eighty percent of the time without surgery or toxic treatments. We can help terminal cases die with dignity and minimal suffering. And we can strengthen people who've been treated for cancer and probably prevent its reccurence. In fact I've never seen a recurrence of cancer in someone we've treated. . . . But we don't treat cancer at Hahnemann Clinic."

"Why not?"

"Because in California, non-toxic treatment of cancer is illegal! It's the damn law. In California the only legal treatment for cancer—by *any* physician—is radiation, surgery and chemotherapy —all of which are poisonous or violently destructive to the body."

"What about other states?"

"In every other state, cancer can be and is being treated successfully by homeopaths. But in California we have to wait until the damage has been done and the cancer has been removed or poisoned. For people who can't leave the state, I'm forced to recommend surgery, then offer to help them pick up the pieces with homeopathy."

"That must be hard to do."

"Damn hard, because the toxic treatments don't cure and they often weaken or kill the patient! But the malpractice liability is enormous for any doctor who doesn't play the game, homeopaths included. Nothing the patient can sign can protect you from the wrath, anger, guilt and grief of relatives who decide old Aunt May was killed by this quack homeopath."

"Are there skilled homeopaths in other states who can treat cancer victims?"

"Sure. The IFH will provide the names of classical homeopaths in other parts of the country."

AIDS

"Most of what I've said about cancer also applies to homeopathic treatment of AIDS. When we get an AIDS patient early we can cure him over half the time, providing he cooperates. In more advanced cases the cure rate goes down. And when the patient is terminal we can offer him valuable palliative treatment."

"So it's not against the law in California to treat AIDS?"

"That's open to question. Some AIDS cases *are* a kind of cancer. But I do treat AIDS. Many homeopaths don't. The cancer law hasn't been applied to AIDS yet because allopathy hasn't come up with any kind of halfway successful AIDS treatment. When and if it does, it will probably invoke the law to protect itself against the 'quacks,' meaning anyone who tries to help who is viewed as competition. I take AIDS cases because homeopathy can help and even cure, and because there's such a desperate need."

"How many AIDS cases have you treated so far?"

"More than two dozen."

"How many of them did you help?"

"Most of them—until the patients took drugs and antidoted their remedy. Seven or eight patients have antidoted, but they're still with me and I'm trying to get them back on track and headed again toward a cure. Then there are the terminal cases who hear about me too late. They usually die in a week or so. The rest we can usually cure or help."

"Is there a lot of demand?"

"Too much. Until recently I was getting one, two and sometimes three new patients a week—mostly referrals from San Francisco's gay community. I don't know what I'll do if the demand keeps up. Having so many potentially fatal cases is a strain. And it takes considerable experience with constitutional prescribing to be successful with AIDS. We have to get them at an early stage and they have to be willing to radically change their lifestyles."

"What changes do you require?"

"What we ask is really minimal, but for many it's too much. They're not used to being asked for self-discipline or self-denial, because allopathy makes no such demands. They have to remain celibate, go on a good diet, and give up drugs of all kinds, otherwise they're wasting my time and theirs. It took me awhile to learn that some of them take Butyl nitrate to enhance orgasms. 'Poppers' they're called. Now that I'm hip, I warn them that they have to give up poppers if they want my help. They swear they won't touch them, but some of them probably will, and when they do they'll blow it for both of us. It's a shame."

"So, for now you're not worried about the law?"

"Right. For now I'm willing to take a chance with highly motivated, early-stage cases, because I know I can help, maybe even save their lives. But AIDS relatives are even more likely to be volatile because the patients are promiscuous and gay. Potentially that makes for extra anger and guilt on the part of the relatives. But I'm willing right now to take the risk because there *is* no allopathic alternative."

Heart Disease

"We can cure heart disease in its early stages, providing it's safe to take the patient off medication. Many heart patients are taking drugs that will antidote the homeopathic remedy. Often they've been taking them for years. Most of the time they don't need them. The allopaths who put them on the drugs are just afraid to take them off, because if something happens they might be sued. So they leave them on ... forever. But once in a while there's a case where it's life-or-death dangerous to stop medication. We can't treat those cases.

"Do any laws govern treatment?"

"No, but malpractice liability does. To avoid being sued, you usually have to put the patient in the hospital, where they are quickly given allopathic drugs, and the drugs antidote the remedy, canceling the treatment."

"So the hospital is the problem?"

"That and the allopathic drugs. When I was a brand new homeopath I attended a conference where a woman in the audience had a heart attack. She didn't want to go to the hospital, so she was treated homeopathically by the faculty members right in her hotel room. All the pain and congestive failure and everything else were cured on the spot."

"That was it?"

"Right. Another time, I was moonlighting in an emergency room in Sebastopol when an alcoholic with a ruined liver and kidneys came in. He'd just had a heart attack. We put him in the intensive care unit. His x-rays showed his lungs were almost completely filled with fluid. Because his organs couldn't take it, we didn't give him drugs. Instead, I treated him homeopathically. A couple of hours later, an x-ray showed that his lungs were completely clear. The next day he felt fine and walked out of the hospital in a huff because they wouldn't let him smoke." He chuckled.

"What did you give him?"

"Arnica, although the resident radiologist was convinced it was digitalis.... So we can treat heart disease effectively and usually without the need of hospitalization, But the social and legal complications can be tricky. Our cure rate goes up if we catch the problem early."

Hypertension

"We can cure high blood pressure, but, again, allopathic drugs antidote our remedies. In the vast majority of cases, hypertension patients are being over-treated with drugs, even by modern allopathic standards. Studies show the morbidity rate is actually higher in cases of moderate high blood pressure treated with drugs than in similar cases not being treated at all. So it's often not too hard to get those people off drugs. But if the blood pressure is *extremely* high, it may be dangerous to stop drugs. So *no* patient should ever stop taking any kind of drug on his own. That decision should always be governed by a doctor."

"So hypertension medicines tend to do more harm than good?"

"Right ... in moderate hypertension. I saw a patient today who originally came to me with high blood pressure. She was taking medication, but her blood pressure was 180/100. The medication wasn't helping, so I had her stop and gave her a homeopathic remedy. Right away her blood pressure dropped to normal. It's now stabilized at 130/85. Before we take anyone off medication we take their cases in great detail, including possible inherited susceptibilities."

"Is the homeopathic cure rate for hypertension also around 80 percent?"

"Yes, but we look at the problem individually. We're primarily interested in freeing the patient of symptoms and risks. We're less concerned with numbers than the allopaths. We're not concerned if the blood pressure reading is high, as long as it's not affecting the body. People don't realize that the *normal* range of blood pressure varies considerably among individuals. Some people are perfectly healthy with moderately high readings. In those cases we don't try to bring it down."

"Don't fix what ain't broke!"

"Exactly!"

Arthritis

"The vast majority of arthritis cases are treatable homeopathically. We don't have much trouble getting people off drugs, and we cure about eighty percent of our cases. If it's early we have a much better chance. If there's a lot of joint deformity the cure rate goes down. We can't reverse extensive mechanical damage. And there are rare incurable cases of arthritis that we can't help."

"Arthritis is systemic?"

"Yep, systemic and miasmatic, requiring constitutional treatment. So it's a long slow process. We can't cure overnight. It takes time to bring the body back—several years in a high percentage of cases. Remember, when I say eighty percent cures, that means twenty percent failures. Some cases are incurable."

Alzheimer's Disease

"Alzheimer's is a hard one because it's relatively new and not promptly diagnosed. Usually by the time we're asked to treat Alzheimer's, the case is too far advanced. My experience under those circumstances is bad. I don't get good results. I'm sure that we could cure it if we got cases at an early stage."

"So the problem is early diagnosis?"

"As far as identification goes, yes. Actually, we probably treat Alzheimer's all the time without recognizing it as such. We often see people who are 'prematurely senile,' along with other problems, and we can usually cure their mental plane problems. The memory improves and their forgetfulness goes away, but it's just part of their overall symptom picture. And it never gets diagnosed as Alzheimer's."

Neurological Disorders

"It's the same with Parkinson's Disease or Multiple Sclerosis—or ALS (Lou Gherig's Disease) or *any* of those neurological disorders. If we get them early enough, we can cure them. But if the stage is advanced, there's enough damage to the neurons themselves that we can't overcome it. We can't repair the damage to the cells beyond a certain point. I think it will turn out to be the same with Alzheimer's, when we gain more experience. Research is showing that there's a lot of deformity in the neurons in Alzheimer's, and it's probably irreversible for mechanical reasons. That's why we don't get results. The same is true with a real advanced case of Parkinson's, and that's why we can't cure it."

"Can you clarify that?"

"In a lot of these crippling diseases there are mechanical effects on the body. In multiple sclerosis, for instance, the nerve sheaths decay. In rheumatoid arthritis the joints decay. In Parkinson's Disease there's substantia nigra destruction in the brain. This mechanical destruction finally interrupts body function irreversibly. As a general rule, we can cure these conditions for the first eight or ten years. That's George Vithoulkas' rule of thumb. My experience backs it up, depending on how much medication has been given to suppress it. The greater the suppression, the more difficult the treatment."

"What about after eight years?"

"It's worth a try, even with the deepest cases—with the understanding that there won't be a total cure. If the condition is difficult or impossible to reverse, we can still probably arrest the degeneration. I've got quite a few cases where we stopped the degeneration and the condition has been stabilized for years. That's the best that can be done."

Obesity and Baldness

"The drug industry spends billions in hopes of finding cures for baldness and obesity because there's big money in vanity-oriented cosmetic drugs. With the allopathic approach, you have to take a drug for each separate symptom, and usually you have to keep taking it forever. That generates billions of dollars in profits. The whole allopathic approach is designed to maximize the sale of expensive drugs. When I quit conventional medicine and started looking for an alternative, I began to see the drug industry's pernicious influence on our thinking. It came to me in a revelation."

"What happened?"

"I was walking one day across a lawn, when I asked myself, 'What if ordinary lawn clippings turned out to cure cancer? What if that was a fact of the universe? What would happen? Would a cheap cure be developed?' The answer is, 'Hell, no!' The drug industry would discredit it as quackery, like they did Laetrile. A cheap cure would threaten the industry to its very core. The people who run the drug companies would do *any*thing to suppress it.

"But these are the same people who support and control all our medical schools. When I realized that, it dawned on me that my medical training was based on the drug industry's political and financial dynamics, not on healing. I realized that my whole medical training was suspect! It was a profound discovery, and it made me reconsider all the healing alternatives that had been branded in medical school as heresy and quackery.

"Getting back to the subject, we're very poor at treating moderate obesity. It's a lifestyle problem, not a manifestation of disease.

We won't even try. But we *can* effectively treat extreme obesity, the so-called 'glandular' cases.... Ordinary male baldness is not homeopathically treatable, because it's not a disease. And I've never seen constitutional treatment start hair growing again. By the way, I'd beware the new drugs that stimulate new hair growth in the follicles. There may be substantial side effects."

Arteriosclerosis

"That's not exactly a disease in our view, although it *can* cause strokes and heart attacks that lead to death. Typically it ravages people in their fifties, sixties and seventies. It's part of the aging process and everyone is susceptible to it. Hardening of the arteries is encouraged by lifestyles that are weak on healthy diet and exercise."

"Can homeopathy help?"

"Yes, we can delay the onset of symptoms by literally decades. Lifelong homeopathic patients, as a general population, live into their seventies, eighties and nineties. We can't stop arteriosclerosis overnight, but over the years constitutional treatment of the whole person will prevent or delay it's occurrence during aging."

High Cholesterol

"High cholesterol is not a disease in itself. I know that people go to health fairs and get themselves tested. Then they start to worry because they're told their cholesterol level is 'above normal.' In homeopathy we aren't bound by 'normal' figures based on population averages. We're concerned with individuals. What's normal for a given individual may not be in the so-called 'normal' range. It's the same as with blood pressure or hemoglobin levels."

"But can homeopathy bring it down?"

"I'd have to say 'no.' We wouldn't treat it by itself. We view high cholesterol as just one symptom out of the whole picture. We treat the whole picture, the whole organism, not just one symptom. Sometimes we see people who have high cholesterol because of their hereditary background, but that doesn't mean those individuals are diseased or even unhealthy. But high cholesterol levels do tend to come down in people we treat holistically."

Diabetes

"As a general rule, we can't cure Juvenile Diabetes, also called Insulin Dependent Diabetes. I don't know exactly why. When we try, we don't ever attempt to reduce insulin dependency. Since the disease destroys a portion of the pancreas, the patient needs insulin to keep from dying. Again, it's the mechanical damage we can't reverse. Incidentally, insulin is just about the only drug that doesn't antidote homeopathic remedies. So diabetes patients needn't fear that we'll try to take it away ... or that it will prevent effective homeopathic treatment of other problems."

"So there's some good news along with the bad?"

"Right. And here's more good news. Although we can't cure Juvenile Diabetes, we *can* cure certain so-called side effects that people associate with it, like the loss of peripheral nerve function, or loss of kidney function or vision. Those things we can treat effectively. I've cured neuropathy and retinopathy in diabetics. So I guess you could say we can cure everything in diabetes except the insulin dependency."

"What about other types of diabetes?"

"The most common form is Maturity Onset Diabetes. It's not a disease, so we don't treat it. It's brought on by obesity, bad diet and not enough exercise. The condition is allopathically treated orally with hypoglycemic agents."

Anorexia

"In the early stages we get dramatic cures, but if the condition has lasted for decades it's very hard to cure. I don't know why because it's not primarily a mechanical problem like those we've been discussing. But it lies very deep and I've found it very difficult to cure. Deep seated anorexia is a real challenge."

That's merely a sample of what constitutional homeopathy can do for the prominent chronic conditions of our time. Virtually *all* chronic conditions are susceptible to homeopathic treatment. It is commonly said in homeopathy that "there are no incurable diseases, only incurable people."

In that respect, there are some limitations. As can be seen from Bill's comments, the earlier the stage, the higher the rate of cure. And, the greater the suppression (from allopathic drugs), the more difficult the homeopathic cure. Homeopathy cannot heal people whose pathology has progressed mechanically to permanent, organic structural changes. And it cannot save people from their ruinous lifestyles. Aside from these limitations, homeopathy can and does cure a very high percentage of patients who cooperate with skilled professional prescribers.

Other Treatable Maladies

There is homeopathic help for all infant and childhood ailments, for female problems of all kinds, from infectious diseases, from epidemics of every sort, from autoimmune and neurological disorders, from any kind of allergy and chronic disease, for accident and injury victims, for mental and psychological problems of every stripe and severity. As we have seen, homeopathy extends readily to veterinary science . . . and dentistry.

Some of the above afflictions are easily curable by lay prescribers or by the patient himself. All he or she needs is a kit and a book or two on home prescribing. These are "acute conditions," defined as those which the body could probably overcome on its own. Deeply entrenched chronic or "constitutional conditions" require the skill and experience of a professional classically trained prescriber.

The distinction between the two classes of ailments (acute and chronic) need not concern the patient. He probably can't hurt himself with low potency homeopathic medicines. If he treats himself with several likely remedies and the condition persists or returns, it probably means that a deeply seated chronic condition exists that will require skilled prescribing. At this point he should seek a well-trained homeopath.

Colds and Flus

I cannot resist a few comments on the so-called "common cold," because the public is daily bombarded on televison with slick high-powered advertising that glibly pictures colds as "incurable."

They're not. But the TV viewer is expected to be grateful that he can purchase an array of expensive medicines that "temporarily relieve" a cold's hateful symptoms. One company likes to advise the public, "Until there's a cure there's...."

Some of the most heavily advertised of these products have been found by the conservative Federal Food and Drug Administration (FDA) to contain "ingredients lacking evidence of safety or effectiveness." Public Citizen's book *Over the Counter Pills That Don't Work* reports that Anacin, Listerine Mouthwash, Nyquil, Preparation H, Excedrin, Dristan tablets, Scope Mouthwash, Robitussin Cough Syrup and Sinutab were all branded by the FDA in 1981 as lacking in safety or effectiveness. But their combined retail sales that year were over half a billion dollars!

The rest of the major over-the-counter (OTC) medicines aren't much better. The only safe and effective ingredient in most of them, according to the FDA, is aspirin or acetaminophen. That list includes Alka Seltzer, Anacin, Bufferin, Cope, Datril, Excedrin, Percogesic and Tylenol. An estimated 300,000 OTC drugs have been concocted to tempt suffering viewers, but they're made from only about 1000 different ingredients. And less than a third of these ingredients are rated safe and effective for their intended use by the FDA! The markup on these mostly inexpensive ingredients is astronomical.

How did the drug industry respond to FDA condemnation? Did it take its worthless or harmful products off the market out of concern for the public welfare? Of course not. To combat the bad publicity, it stepped up its advertising to saturation levels, presenting ads that range from misleading to downright fraudulent. The drug pundits know that TV advertising works, and they don't mind robbing the suffering public. These X-rated medicines are still household names, all of them in the top forty in terms of sales. They make up a hefty part of a $10 billion a year business in OTC drugs sold to TV-watching sufferers who vainly hope they will work as promised.

Despite its negative ratings, the sluggish FDA can't bear to crack down on its good friends in the drug industry by actually banning every one of these unsafe or ineffective OTC medicines. It prefers to violate drug laws by allowing the ingredients in these drugs to remain on the market!

Meanwhile, unknown to the general public, there are literally hundreds of safe, cheap, homeopathic remedies that genuinely *cure*, not just *relieve*, cold symtpoms, of every sort ... cough, earache, sleeplessness, stuffy nose, headache, sneezing, sore throat, diarrhea, fever, chills—and every other common symptom you can name. And they do it decisively, fast and without side effects—literally for pennies per dose.

All you have to do is match—or get a homeopath to match—your individual symptom picture to that of the appropriate remedy. If you have a homeopathic kit (costing $40–60 for 30–40 remedies) and a book on diagnosis, you needn't spend a penny or even leave the comfort of your home to get unbelievable and permanent relief.

If you think your family physician cares more about healing you than making money or protecting his status, try asking him what he knows about the effectiveness of homeopathic remedies. Chances are 10 to 1 you'll encounter one of the following reactions: anger, ignorance, prejudice, dismissal, irritation, defensiveness, disdain, ridicule, apathy, condescension, condemnation or something similar. If I'm right, ask yourself if your doctor sounds like a healer ... someone who truly wants to end suffering?

Chances are he'll change the subject and slide open a drawer full of free samples from his benefactors in the drug industry and tell you, more or less, that "the doctor knows best," and what's best for you is somewhere in his drawer. He has to believe that—or pretend to—or his world would collapse. If you think what's in that drawer is good for you or will benefit your body, consider a few random statistics that reflect allopathic health care (i.e. the doctors and the drug industry). Chronic disease is steeply on the rise, and it disables younger people every year. In a vain attempt to get relief, Americans consume 20,000 tons of aspirin every year. Some 200,000 cancer patients are annually poisoned with chemotherapy.

Two million Americans are afflicted with Alzheimer's, a disease unknown a few years ago. Twenty percent of the patients released by the hospital are forced to return within two months.

And more than a third of hospital beds are occupied by doctor-induced (iatrogenic) illness.

Conventional drugs may be temporarily helpful in relieving pain, but they rarely cure and often do more harm than good ... not to mention the side effects. As evidence of this trend, the FDA gets substantially more reports of adverse reactions every year. Consider a comparison of allopathic drugs and homeopathic remedies. New drugs by the hundreds are introduced each year with great fanfare ... in hopes that they'll sell. Meanwhile, hundreds more are quietly withdrawn because they didn't sell, proved ineffective or caused dangerous or intolerable side effects.

In contrast, *all* of the homeopathic remedies in use during Hahnemann's time are still safe and effective—200 years later! They're all approved by the FDA, cause no adverse reactions, and don't need to be "new and improved" every year. They just work. That says something about which branch of medicine is most effective and most scientific?

Deaths from heart disease run 600,000 a year and coronary bypass surgery, the principal allopathic answer, is rapidly increasing —up from 50,000 bypasses in 1977 to over 200,000 in 1986. As many as 90 percent of these operations, it has been estimated, would be unnecessary if doctors fully informed their patients about programs of diet and exercise.

Surgery, says the homeopath, should be a last resort, but with allopaths it often comes first ... because they have no effective, safe medicines to offer. Homeopathic remedies, on the other hand, are so effective that they usually make surgery unnecessary in, for instance, curing breast and ovarian cysts, uterine fibroids, enlarged thyroid, kidney stones, gallstones, chronically swollen tonsils and adenoids. And recurrent vaginal bleeding can be cured homeopathically without a hysterectomy.

Homeopaths—and other sensible physicians—prefer to try mild, safe, non-toxic, non-invasive remedies before resorting to surgery and toxic drugs. That's no more than common sense and respect for human suffering!

Tens of millions of patients have experienced beneficial results, without side effects, from homeopathic remedies. And many of them have been permanently and completely cured. Homeopaths are used to hearing their patients say, "I never felt better in my life!"

Homeopathic Dentistry

Next comes a look at a so-called "homeopathic dentist." My Echo neighbor Jeanne told me a dentist describing himself as a homeopath insisted that the source of her chronic nasal congestion was Mercury poisoning from the silver amalgam fillings in her teeth. He had discovered this, he claimed, by measuring her imbalances on a Dermatron machine, which also told him which homeopathic remedy would restore her body's energy balance.

She gave him the go-ahead and one by one he removed her silver fillings and replaced them with gold—at considerable expense. He told her it would be approximately a year before she received benefits from the removal of the silver. I told Bill the story and asked what he thought.

"I think it's baloney! The machine is supposed to measure the flow of energy in the meridians and diagnose chemical deficiencies in the body. I tried that 'remove the Mercury' strategy back in the early seventies on half a dozen patients—including myself—and found it worthless. All of us had all our fillings replaced. It cost each of us two thousand dollars and it failed in every single case. Not one of us got the slightest benefit."

"Then why do people do it? Why did you?"

"Because it sounds good in theory. Different metals *do* produce an electric current that might easily be harmful. And the constant presence of Mercury *could* be constantly poisoning the body. Since Mercury is a remedy for hay fever, if the excess Mercury is removed, the hay fever should go away. It sounds good, but I've never seen it work."

"What do you think of this machine?"

In measuring the flow of electric current across the patient's meridians, it produces a lot of untestable hypotheses. The main problem is the assumption that all the meridians ought to be firing at the same energy rate, like spark plugs in a car. Who's to say the 'imbalance' the machine reveals isn't the natural state of affairs in that individual? As I understand the body, it's in a fluid state, constantly changing in order to deal with stress and avoid producing symptoms. In my experience, patients treated on the basis of machine findings usually get worse on the mental and emotional planes and experience a drop in energy!"

"So you condemn the practice of switching fillings."

"No," he chuckled. "Not entirely. But the diagnosis should be made by a genuine homeopath, not some dentist with a machine. The approach may be valid if the patient is known to be sensitive to Mercury. I just had the fillings replaced in one of my patients, a lady with Parkinson's Disease, because her remedy picture is Mercury, and Mercury is the major remedy for Parkinson's. We agonized and debated a long time before I sent her to the dentist, because she hasn't a lot of money. But we weren't making progress and I thought maybe the fillings in her teeth were holding us back."

"Did it help?"

"Preliminary results are zero, but maybe in time it will help. If switching fillings works at all, it should help in this case—providing her fillings are part of the problem. We'll just have to wait and see. Let me know what luck your friend Jeanne has. If neither case gets better, we may have to junk this approach."

Insanity

Finally, I asked Bill what homeopathy can do for the so-called "insane," patients relegated to spending the rest of their lives heavily drugged in crowded mental hospitals.

"We are perfectly capable of curing psychotic conditions like schizophrenia, manic-depressive psychosis, suicidal depression and so forth constitutionally," he said, "if we have the needed facilities, mainly hospitals. Our only problem is patient management. Most of these people are kept sedated and out of trouble with major allopathic tranquilizers. To treat them homeopathically, we have to take them off drugs because tranquilizers dependably antidote our remedies. That requires a hospital, which we don't have—yet."

"With a homeopathic hospital you could cure mental illness?"

"Absolutely. With a hospital and staff we could cure the mentally disabled in droves. But mental conditions that aren't danger-ous—depression, insomnia, anxieties, phobias and all kinds of neu-roses—those we cure routinely. And our cure rate is high. We can also cure early stage schizophrenics and manic-depressives who aren't yet a threat. After all, we cure mental afflictions routinely in most constitutional cases. Mental and emotional symptoms figure prominently, as you know, in all homeopathic diagnosis."

"So it's just a matter of degree?"

"Right. Mental patients are just sicker than most people. If the focus is on the mental plane, the patient usually has a weak vital force. These people tend to be layered cases and antidote easily, but their extreme behavior makes correct remedy selection fairly easy. Cures aren't quick and easy, but our success rate is high with manageable mental patients. And we'll do just as well with violent cases when we have the facilities and staff to treat them."

Hopefully this brief survey of what homeopathy can cure will help the reader assess the chances of curing the varied ills of family and friends.

17

Gellie's Constitutional

... and My Second Year Test in the Desert

It was September twenty-first, the last day of summer, when I descended to the desert for the acid test. The rabbit brush was blooming but the sage hadn't opened. I felt strong and confident. This was to be my second year examination. Bill had predicted that I'd be, "more than fifty percent better" this second pollen season, and just three months before he'd confirmed that I was right on schedule.

So I tried not to think about allergy symptoms. It wasn't until the third day that I began to sneeze and blow my nose. But after a few minutes my body would recover and the episode would end. On the fifth day we returned to the cabin to finish closing for the winter. In the pollen-free mountains my hay fever vanished. When we returned to Walker the sage had finally opened! Now came the real test!

After twelve hours my eyes began to water and I braced myself for the onslaught, but after a few minutes my symptoms went away. Over the next few days a familiar pattern emerged: unpredictable ups and downs reminiscent of my adventures with the isopathic remedy. As long as I stayed inside I was fine, but after playing basketball on the windy outdoor court, I could count on half an hour of sneezing. I felt a little like a yo-yo, falling toward the depths ... then climbing back to comfort, but the overall result was satisfactory. I seemed to have found a symptom plateau—and it was substantially higher than on the previous year with the isopathic remedy.

After four days with the sage I was back in Berkeley, reporting to Bill. He was pleased. "I'd say you're doing fine. And next year your symptoms should be very insignificant."

When I told him about the deluge of pine pollen at Echo that had opened old sores on my face, he said, "Don't worry. Tuberculinums are 'better with pine.' But that also means you're sensitive to it. You just got a toxic dose. Forget it." He leaned back in his chair. "No, the only question now is, 'How long will the remedy continue to act?' If it wears off, we give you another dose. If it doesn't, then year by year you'll just keep getting better. You can call anytime, but essentially I'm discharging you from treatment."

That was welcome news, but somehow shocking, too. "What about my chances of anitdoting?" I asked. "You quoted George as saying a remedy that's been working two years can't be anitdoted."

"In my experience it's *three* years, but once it's set you won't relapse again. It's a little like the setting of concrete. Concrete at first is weak and easy to crack. But gradually it gets harder until finally it's the same as rock. In the first few months, homeopathic remedies are easily antidoted. One cup of coffee will do it. But as time goes by it takes more and more ... until finally it won't antidote at all."

On that note our doctor-patient relationship came to an end. When I returned to the desert two days later, my symptoms were all but gone. And they troubled me very little during the final two days as we packed for our winter migration to Hawaii.

Back on the Big Island we settled into old routines, but Gellie caught one cold after another. One evening we sat listening to muffled coughs from her bedroom. Deanne frowned. "I've tried Aconite and Pulsatilla, but nothing clears her up. She gets sick too easily. Maybe it's time for a constitutional."

I agreed. A constitutional at age eight could reduce future suffering, make way for greater happiness and add a decade to her lifespan. Gellie played so hard that she often wore herself out. If we didn't limit the stress in her life, she dependably got sick. So we decided to ask Michael Traub to take her case. A few days later he arrived about sunset and we gathered in the living room. I offered him a beer, but he said he'd wait til we were done. He sat on the couch, I took a chair, and Deanne cooked dinner within earshot in the kitchen. Gellie sat down on a low swivel stool facing Michael. They had never met.

"Your name is Angela, but they call you Gellie?" he asked, smiling.

She nodded, idly swiveling from side to side as she sized him up. Our little blond girl wasn't overawed by adults, and she liked being the center of attention.

"Why are your mommy and dad having you talk with me tonight?"

"Because I wasn't feeling so good."

"What was wrong?"

"I was having headaches and coughs. And sniffles. And a stuffy nose. And a sore throat."

How long have you been having these? A couple weeks? Couple months? Couple years?"

"I don't know.... A couple weeks, I guess."

"What about today? Have you felt sick today?"

"When I woke up this morning I felt yucky ... with a headache ... and the sniffles."

"The stuff coming out of your nose ... was it thick and yellow or watery?"

She thought about that. "Watery," she decided.

Michael nodded and made some notes on the clipboard in his lap. Then he turned to us. "Okay, mommy and daddy, we need some help."

Deanne was ready. "This morning when she woke up she complained of a headache and didn't want to go to school. The headaches come periodically, whether she's sick or not. She comes home from school and says she had a headache or feels dizzy. And usually there's nothing else wrong with her."

"It's the same thing with her cough," I added. "As soon as she and I start wrestling, she starts coughing." I turned to Gellie. "Right baby?"

She soberly nodded.

"What's it like when you get dizzy?" Michael asked her.

She revolved her head and rolled her eyes dramatically. "I feel like the room's going around!"

"Does it only happen at school?"

"Sometimes when I'm doing my homework, too."

"It isn't just when she's concentrating," Deanne corrected. "She was often dizzy last summer at Echo."

Michael nodded. "Is the dizziness bad enough to make her stop and sit down?"

"Not very often. She's a demon for play," I said. "She doesn't ever want to stop."

"What brings on your headaches?" he asked Gellie.

"When the kids are really noisy. When they bother me."

"It isn't always noise," Deanne reminded her. "This morning you said you had a headache when you woke up. And it wasn't noisy at all."

"Sounds like the dizziness and headaches are chronic," said Michael, "while the other stuff's acute." He turned to Angela. "Do you like school?"

She nodded vigorously.

"Do you get good grades?"

"A's and B's."

"Any behavioral problems at school?" he asked us. "Anything her teacher complains about?"

Deanne and I looked at one another. We'd had a conference with her teacher just the day before. "Her teacher says she can't stand anyone close to her or touching her or in front of her," I reported. "She's hypersensitive that way. We've heard it from all her teachers. She overreacts, bitterly complaining, sometimes crying. A week ago she came to me after school very upset because a boy had put his arm on her desk."

"Why did that upset you?" Michael asked her.

"He was putting it right where I was trying to write a word!" she said indignantly.

"What did you do?"

"I told the teacher," she said righteously.

"Is she something of a tattletale?" he asked us.

Deanne nodded. "She gets upset when people don't do 'right.' She gets mad over things that have nothing to do with her. And she's very emotional about it."

"Her teachers also say she's bossy," I added. "We scold her but it doesn't seem to help. She has to be the leader. She tells everybody what to do. But somehow she gets away with it. The kids do what she says . . . and come back for more."

"She's very emotional," Deanne put in. "She cries very easily." She told how she'd accidentally pulled the tassels out of Gellie's twirling baton with the vacuum. "I couldn't believe how she carried on. She cried and cried and cried. And she wouldn't accept my apology . . . even though she hadn't touched that baton in six months!"

"The decoration was gone!" Gellie pouted.

"When she gets upset," asked Michael, "how does she respond to consolation?"

"Oh, she *loves* it," said Deanne.

"Here's another paradox," I told him. "While she's confident and aggressive socially, she's very timid physically. She's way behind the other kids in roller skating, swimming and riding a bike—even though we've pushed her to learn."

"She just won't take any risks," said Deanne.

"Generally she minds well," I went on. "But she refuses to do what she's told during swimming lessons. Her fear seems bigger than her trust of us."

"So, in some ways she's very venturesome, and in other ways very timid," Michael summed up. He turned to look in a book. Gellie seized the opportunity to slide off the stool and climb on my back, giggling. Deanne told her to go back and sit down. She cheerfully obeyed.

"Why are you afraid to swim?" Michael asked her.

She swung on the stool. "I'm not afraid in the shallow water, but I'm scared where I can't touch."

"Why? Do you think your parents would let you drown?"

She nodded without hesitation.

"Really? No, they wouldn't let you drown!"

She giggled but wouldn't change her story.

"What about roller skating?"

"I can skate," she assured him.

"What about riding a bike? Are you afraid of that?"

"Not any more."

"But you were?"

She nodded. "I was afraid of getting hurt."

Deanne told about the day she ran her bike into a car at the other end of the parking lot. "She was so afraid it would happen again that she refused to ride down there. I worked on her for days! Finally I told her, 'You're not getting off that bicycle until you ride all the way down to the end and back. Finally she did it.

Apparently undismayed, Gellie was pretending to ride a bicycle, holding imaginary handlebars, leaning as she banked the turns. Michael smiled. "I see she has a good imagination."

"She does," said Deanne. "And she likes to entertain people. She's very pleasant to be around. When you punish her she gets over it quickly. She doesn't sit around and mope. Teachers basically like her because she tries hard to please and is pleasant and outgoing."

I nodded. "She has a very sunny disposition."

Gellie sat down on the couch beside Michael to see what he was writing. "Daddy, look how much he wrote about me," she said excitedly.

Michael stopped and turned to her. "What else are you afraid of?"

"Nightmares ... about haunted houses ... and people getting killed, about monsters and witches."

"What else?"

She thought a moment. "Getting hurt. Breaking my arm ... or my leg. Falling off a high roof. Or if my friends are getting mad at me and hitting me with sticks."

"What about the dark? Does it scare you?"

"Not any more," said Deanne. "Not since we convinced her there aren't any monsters or ghosts."

Gellie laughed.

"What are your favorite foods? he asked her.

"Spaghetti and macaroni and cheese ... and mushrooms and pizza. And ice cream." She giggled. "And candy! Yum!"

"Do you like salt on your food?"

"Salt. Blaaaah!"

"How about spicy things ... like hot sauce?"

"Yuck."

"How's her thirst?"

"She likes cold water," said Deanne. "But she forgets to drink. She's too busy playing."

"Any bad reactions to foods?"

"Ice cream or a lot of milk stuffs up her nose," said Deanne.

"Does she sleep through the night?"

We nodded.

"Does she do anything unusual in her sleep? Walk? Talk? Cry? Grind her teeth?"

"No. She kicks off the covers and she sprawls all over the bed in crazy positions, but mostly on her back."

Gellie got the giggles.

"What illnesses has she had?"

"Chicken pox, measles."

"Any broken bones? Was she ever in the hospital?"

"No, never."

He wrote for a while before asking, "So her major chronic symptoms are the headaches and dizziness? Anything else?"

"Whenever she's under stress," said Deanne, "she gets a cold or a cough."

"Any cold sores? Or warts? Or digestive problems?"

"Yes," said Deanne. "Sometimes after dinner she'll say her stomach hurts."

"Does she sweat much?" Before we could reply he asked Gellie for her hand to check for sweaty palms. Her hand was dry.

"She's a good eater," Deanne volunteered. "She eats almost anything you give her.... Angela, is there anything you really dislike?"

"I *hate* stir fry!"

Michael turned to Gellie. "Is there anything else I should

know about you? Anything that's been left out? Anything you'd like to tell me?"

She shook her head.

He turned to us. "What would you say is the single most unique thing about Gellie? What makes her special, or different?"

Deanne nodded for me to go first. "My vote would go to her cheerfulness."

Michael looked at Deanne.

"I was going to say the same thing. She's a very pleasant child to be around. People gravitate toward her. Kids come from all over the village to play with her, and she organizes them all. She pulls them into her fantasies. She makes up these games and the rules change every thirty seconds. The kids sometimes look puzzled, but they do what she tells them. They let her boss them around."

Michael leaned back and put away his clipboard. "Okay," he smiled. "I'm ready now for that beer."

After dinner was over and Gellie was tucked in bed, the three of us settled in the shadowy lanai, fanned by a warm breeze. "What constitutional remedy did you come up with for Gellie?" Michael asked Deanne.

"I think she's Pulsatilla ... because she's emotional, warm-blooded, likes the open air and wants to please."

He shook his head. "No, she's not Pulsatilla. They're timid. She's not. With her cheerful disposition and outgoing personality and liking to entertain and fantasizing a lot and being imaginative, her picture is classical Phosphorus. Pulsatillas like consolation, but they don't go after it like Phosphorus does. Phosphorus likes being in the spotlight, being the center of attention. And that's exactly what you were telling me about Gellie. Phosphorus are much more confident of themselves than Pulsatilla. All the strokes she gets, all that popularity and attention, it helps build her confidence."

"She's confident, all right, in a lot of areas," said Deanne, "but she also has her fears ... her unwillingness to take physical risks."

Michael smiled. "Phosphorus is confident in nearly everything they do, but it's also a remedy known for having a lot of fears, especially of monsters and thunderstorms. And they're easily startled, too."

Deanne nodded. "When she was very little she definitely was afraid of thunder and monsters. And she's always complaining that I 'scare' her when I walk in her room unexpectedly."

"The desire for ice cold drinks helped me, too. That's strong in Phosphorus. Some of the food cravings fit Sulphur more than Phosphorus. Sulphur may be an underlying layer. She's very warm, she uncovers, she likes sweets … whereas Phosphorus likes salty things, not sweets. Her desire to be the leader also suggests Sulphur. They don't like to follow others. They want to be in charge. But I don't have any doubts about Phosphorus. The thing that convinced me was your calling her disposition 'sunny' and agreeing that her number one quality was her cheerfulness."

Now that Gellie was taken care of, it was Deanne's turn. Recently she'd experienced a return of her congestion, drainage, the tickle in her throat and the resulting cough … in fact all her pre-homeopathic symptoms. It was a relapse of the sort she'd experienced nine months before. At that time, Michael had given her Arsenicum 1M, the same remedy Bill Gray had given her nine months before. The original dose had been 200.

"If Arsenicum's the right remedy," she asked, "how come it wears off after only nine months? It's happened twice."

"I don't know," said Michael. "It shouldn't. Your symptoms haven't changed. I don't see anything in your picture except Arsenicum. Before we go to a higher potency, let's see what another dose of 1M will do. Then we'll do followups on both you and Gellie in a month."

18

Follow-Up & Finale

... an Update of the Cases of My Family and Friends

It's time to take a farewell look at the principal characters in our story, starting with Jeanne, whose so-called homeopathic dentist had removed all her silver fillings and replaced them with gold, to get rid of a chronic throat problem. Excerpts from two letters tell what happened. In December Jeanne wrote ...

"Not only did my old throat problem begin again when I got home from Echo, Kaiser (Hospital) tells me my cholesterol is still too high! Though I lost 12 pounds since last spring, the Kaiser internist scolded me for not sticking to his low fat diet! As far as the throat goes, they keep saying there's 'no problem.' A fine answer after three years of diagnosis!

"I could hardly wait to get home. I stormed in the door, called Hahnemann and asked for an appointment with Bill Gray. I was surprised I only had to wait two weeks. Well, you were right. It's a wonderful process. I felt like a real person again ... that someone really cared and was asking about my life rather than just surface level symptoms.

"It seems I fit the Natrum muriaticum category. Knowing much from reading your book, I had already given up coffee (a terrible struggle), had my teeth fixed beforehand and banned all camphor from my collection. Mint is also blacklisted for this medicine. It's been five days now since I swallowed the Natrum muriaticum.

Today my throat is a bit more sore and my voice is hoarse again, so the treatment must be working."

In reply I wrote Jeanne, "It was the runaround my mother got from Kaiser that sent her to Hahnemann, too. And she's also Natrum mur! She's gotten considerable benefit—considering that she won't give up her heart medicine or her electric blanket!"

Three months later Jeanne wrote, "My chronic cough and sore larynx were much worse for three weeks. I felt irritable and mourned a lifetime of drinking herb tea, which tasted like rusty pipe water. Had I not been prepared for 'the aggravations,' I probably would have found solace in coffee again."

When the aggravations passed Jeanne found herself changed. "I felt more centered, healthier and purposeful in my life, but my pragmatic self was quick to dismiss homeopathy as hokum, and attribute my improved attitude and health to something more metaphysical, or coincidental. Now I cough very rarely and my throat hasn't been sore for two months. I have lost twelve pounds and over 100 cholesterol points, and I feel tremendous new energy in my life."

My mother reports, "I've got lots of energy. The congestion and drainage are gone, and I'm getting those marvelous feelings of well-being again!"

Peggy tried to get her to cut back on her two heart medicines, to give the remedy a better chance, but Mom refused. It had taken her too long to find the delicate balance that holds the side effects down to mere acid indigestion. For emergencies, she also carries in her purse nitroglycerine (originally a homeopathic remedy) for heart pains and an ounce of vodka for sudden attacks of throat paralysis. Nevertheless, Mom increasingly relies on Peggy and homeopathy for her health care.

From my perspective, her gains have been substantial. Before homeopathy, weakened by radiation therapy, she was catching every bug that came along. She hasn't caught one since. And her voice, which was gravelly and hoarse, is clear and she can sing again. But the change I notice most is in her spirit, her vigor, her fresh outlook on life. She used to hate exercise. Now she flexes with the TV exercise ladies or walks around the block. "Or if it's cold or rainy," she told me proudly, "I walk briskly around the house 25 times."

A year ago when she completed her radiation treatment, she was sent to Kaiser's Cancer Therapy group for a month—to gain support. Instead of quitting when her time was up, she stuck around to help. "I hated all the long faces, that grim atmosphere," she told me, "even if they *were* all dying and in pain. I started with humorous quips about what we go through in the hospital. When that brought smiles, I tried anecdotes, monologues, jokes and funny stories—anything to lift them out of the doldrums."

She still shows up every few weeks, determined to cheer and entertain ... and have herself some fun. After one session an old man, tears in his eyes, gripped her hand tightly as he said, "Thank you for making me laugh again!"

The turnover from week to week, Mom tells me, is great, as one after another of her friends succumbs or departs to the hospice to die. But Mom doesn't let it bother her. "I go there to laugh. Being silly and making people laugh makes me happy too. I never knew I had such a sense of humor."

Before homeopathy she didn't!

On a recent visit with Bill he gave me a likely glimpse of his future. He had just returned from lecturing in Norway, and Roger and his wife Nancy were just back from giving seminars in Holland. They came home to find a stack of requests for homeopathic teaching from Austria, England, Switzerland, East Germany and Holland again.

"The three of us came up with an exciting idea. Instead of merely presenting what interests us or our sponsors, why not organize ourselves into an international school of homeopathy, with a curriculum taken from our courses here? We could add Jonathan Shore and a couple of classic Vithoulkian teachers from Europe to round out the faculty. Students would get more value from a systematized course of study than they do from random one-shot lectures. When they got through they'd have a sound base for practicing ... and a diploma.

The growing worldwide demand for homeopathic teaching is

very gratifying to Bill. "Our school has only been open five years and already there's international demand for it!"

"Why do they come to you in America, where homeopathy has so long been suppressed?" I asked. "Why don't they turn to professionals in India or Greece?"

"Because they want teachers ... English-speaking, Vithoulkian-trained teachers ... and George is no longer available. (He's holed up to write his own Materia Medica.) Most of those people in Europe and India are just practitioners. They don't teach."

Recently Bill told me, "The suppression of homeopathy in America early in the century could be a blessing in disguise. It's given us the opportunity to start fresh with a clean slate and establish pure classical homeopathy."

A month after Hawaii naturopath Michael Traub came to our house to take Gellie's case and Deanne's, the three of us were in his office for a follow-up. Gellie told him she felt better, but not much more, so he turned to us.

"All her common symptoms are gone," Deanne reported. "except for a little coughing. No more headaches or dizziness or stomach aches. But after about a week she developed rawness and even bleeding around the rim of each nostril. It comes and goes. Calendula made it better but it hasn't gone away."

Michael nodded and peered into Gellie's red-crusted nostrils. "Phosphorus is the primary remedy for nasal bleeding. So this is a confirmatory symptom."

"A proving?" I asked.

"Yes. Phosphorus is specific for nosebleeds. The crust shows that Phosphorus has acted well. When it happens in the course of a general improvement it's a good sign. It probably won't continue. Have you noticed any behavioral changes, changes in temperament?"

We couldn't think of any. He turned to Angela and smiled. "Good work, Gellie. The crust on your nose should soon go away."

Gellie escaped to the waiting room to play and Michael turned to Deanne. It was a month since he'd given her another dose of Arsenicum 1M, after the first had apparently worn off in nine months. She had just taken a full-time teaching job in cool clammy Waimea and she'd always had trouble while teaching.

"I don't think it helped me," Deanne told him. "I got better during Christmas vacation, but the problem hasn't gone away. When we went out last night in the rain I got a tickle in my throat and started coughing. I couldn't stop! And my ears still sometimes hurt or pop."

He meticulously questioned her about her thirst, fever or sweats, worst times of the day or night, etc. Finally he examined her tongue. "Your symptoms are basically the same, still Arsenicum," he told her. "I think it's still your funadmental remedy, but you may need an acute remedy to deal with this cough. We can give you a higher dose ... 10M instead of 1M. Or try to find another remedy." He didn't sound too hopeful about the latter. Deanne decided to try Arsenicum one more time.

Within a week the crust was gone from Gellie's nose. A week later we stopped giving her Phosphorus, and her health remained excellent, with no return of any of her symptoms. And the Arsenicum 10M had the expected effect of clearing up Deanne's symptoms, even when she went back to rainy Waimea to teach.

As for me, I slowly get better and better. My eyesight improves, my congestion fades, my irritation level drops, my generosity grows. I find myself more philosophical, relaxed and content. Not that my life is all milk and honey. One January night I came out of the sea after sunset and stood dripping on the beach, talking to a friend. By the time I got home I was thoroughly chilled. The next morning I awoke with a heavy cold.

Deanne prescribed Aconite 12 every four hours, along with a gram of vitamin C. By the end of the day I felt I wasn't making any progress, so I quit to let the symptom level build before asking Deanne to retake my case. This time she gave me Allium cepa, the onion that had cured my last cold, six months before at Echo. I soon wished I'd stuck with the Aconite and Vitamin C! I erupted into a sneezing fountain that soaked my pillow when I went to bed.

In the morning Deanne patiently tried again. She sent me outdoors to see if I were better or worse in the open air. When I returned to report "better," she gave me her own remedy, Arsenicum 30. The effect was magical and immediate. The fountain dried up as though a valve had been closed. Within an hour the last of my symptoms had disappeared.

On the eighteenth of June—back now on the mainland at the cabin on Echo Lake—we celebrated the third anniversary of my single dose of Tuberculinum. It was now supposed to have set like concrete and no longer be antidotable, but I planned to take no chances.

In September we returned to the house in the desert for the final test. As Bill had predicted more than three years before, I was "nearly symptom free." Only an occasional sneeze reminded me of the allergy that had made life in the desert unbearable in the fall. Strolling by the river, I paused to tap a heavy sheaf of blossoming sage. I watched the tiny cloud of green dust errupt and disappear on the breeze ... and I smiled.

Mentally and emotionally I'm also improving. When I discover new freedoms, they're like unexpected gifts. I've never thought of myself as a fearful person, but looking back I see that all kinds of minor anxieties have simply melted away. I can truthfully say that I'm happier now than I've ever been before. Never have I felt so content with today ... or more eager for tomorrow. My chief goals nowadays are to be a good husband, father, citizen and son. Being a kind responsible human now means more than wealth or career—not that I'll forsake writing or give away my money! My experience has simply re-ordered my priorities, and they feel more comfortable now.

When I look back more than three years—to the man I was before homeopathy—I see someone quite different. My changes, as they happened, were often too gradual to see, but in the sharp focus of retrospect my growth has been profound ... and profoundly satisfying. And the greatest blessings were those that were completely unexpected ... the better breathing, better eyesight and still declining irritation. It isn't necessary, I've discovered, to accept lifelong disabilities. Homeopathy has the magic to help us heal ourselves. And with the freedom that comes from genuine good health, happiness floats within reach.

As Emerson put it, "The first wealth is health." Another wise man wrote, "Happiness lies first of all in health." Now that I've had a taste of real health, I know the fundamental truth of those statements.

Though Bill has officially "discharged" me as a patient, I'm hopelessly hooked on homeopathy. It's become a way of life, a dependable way of staying happy and well. And I find deep satisfaction in revealing the great hope it offers to others. So does Dr. Deanne.

I'll stay in touch with Bill because he's my doctor and my friend ... and because we're interested in one another's future. He has gotten me to where I am today and I'm grateful.

Of course, I still have plenty of room for growth, so I expect, as Bill put it, "to keep on getting better, year by year."

Epilogue

A Final Look

One Year Later . . .

When Michael Traub's Arsenicum 10M failed to provide Deanne lasting benefits, she returned to Bill Gray, who retook her case. This time he prescribed Kali carbonicum 200. We brought Gellie with us because she once again was catching colds. Bill took her case and gave her Lycopodium. She's been healthy as a little horse ever since.

The Kali carb didn't work for Deanne. When she returned to damp Waimea in Hawaii to teach, her drainage and accompanying symptoms all came back. Bill was lecturing in Europe when we came back to California, so we went to see Roger Morrison. He ordered Deanne's symptoms somewhat differently, concluding that she was allergic to some combination of fungus, mildew and dampness in those clammy Hawaii classrooms. He prescribed Dulcamara 200 which promptly stopped her adverse symptoms—although she hasn't been back to Waimea to test it.

On June 18th we celebrated the fourth anniversary of that single magic dose of Tuberculinum. Three months later in the desert, when the rabbit brush and sage came in bloom, its pollen had no discernible effect on me. My once-devastating allergy had been cured!

But the Tuberculinum hasn't stopped working. I'm still receiving its blessings. Just last spring I discovered I no longer needed constant involvement in major creative projects in order to be happy. For the first time in my life, I was content to simply take things as they came. And when summer arrived I found I no longer had to spend every minute at Echo. We took a raft trip down the Grand Canyon in June, traded cabins on another mountain lake in July, and spent two weeks hiking the Yosemite back country in August. To me, these mental changes were welcome newfound freedoms.

I've also had my share of physical adventures, all of which resulted in noteworthy homeopathic solutions. Last winter, Deanne and I were hiking the empty southern coast of Hawaii when I slipped and fell, landing full force on my face on rock. As always Deanne was carrying her tiny first aid kit. She immediately gave me Arnica 200, which cut the pain in half in less than five minutes. When I got to the car she washed my face and daubed my wounds with Hypericum tincture.

During the hour and a half drive to Michael Traub's office, her two further doses of Arnica saved me considerable pain. Michael said he couldn't improve on her first aid and sent us to a surgeon who put a dozen stitches in my forehead. He wiggled my swollen, misshapen nose and pronounced it unbroken. When his nurse offered pain pills, I declined. When she tried to swab my face with an iodine, Deanne stopped her.

Iodine products, she had learned from homeopath Dorothy Shepherd's books, burn and tan the epithelial tissue of the skin, leaving it half dead and vulnerable to infection, a certain hindrance to healing.

Back home, Deanne kept my wounds clean with Hypericum tincture, and kept the scabs and stitches soft and healing with Calendula cerate. When we returned to the surgeon to have the stitches removed, he was impressed by the swiftness of healing and lack of swelling—which he attributed to his consumate skill! Again he tweaked my tender nose and assured me it wasn't broken.

My Frankenstein forehead was completely healed and scarless within two months, thanks to Deanne's Calendula and Hypericum treatments, but my nose was still so tender that I found myself cringing every time Deanne kissed me. "Your nose HAS to be broken," she frowned. "I'm going to give you Symphytum. They call it 'knit-bone.'" After five daily doses of Symphytum 12, the tenderness was gone and I could wiggle my nose without pain. Amazing! Later, Bill said it was one of the best Symphytum cures he'd ever heard of, probably because the nose bones are so small.

Back in California that spring we visited our friend Yon, who apologized for not getting up to greet us. His injured knee was hurting him. X-rays showed a crack and he was scheduled to have a cast put on his leg three days later. Deanne gave him enough Symphytum 12 for five daily doses and urged him to postpone his visit to the doctor. Yon grew up in Denmark, where he'd known homeopathy, so he readily agreed. At the end of five days the crack in his knee was completely healed, so he canceled his date with the doctor.

Last fall, following a minor shoulder bump in a basketball game, I began to lose mobility in my left arm. In the excitement of a 40-day visit to New Zealand, I nearly forgot about the problem. But when we returned to Hawaii in the spring, I was shocked to find I couldn't swim! Use of my left arm was much too restricted. Michael Traub diagnosed chronic bursitis and prescribed daily doses of Rhus tox 30, supplemented with exercises.

After four days I began to feel exceedingly strange. I thought I must be coming down with some dread New Zealand flu, or suffering a letdown from the rigors of our trip. I ached all over and my appetite was gone. I couldn't reach Michael on the weekend, so unfortunately I kept taking the Rhus tox.

By Monday I felt horrible. Over the telephone Michael diagnosed a Rhus tox "proving." Due to a misunderstanding I'd overdosed on Rhus tox to the point of toxicity. Now I was experiencing the symptoms that it both produced and cured. It was a week and a half before the effects wore off. The experience left me with new respect for the power of potent homeopathic remedies ... and for Samuel Hahnemann and all the dedicated men and women who over the years have taken toxic doses of medicine in order to study the symptoms produced for the benefit of future homeopathic patients.

To avoid the harmless unpleasantness of a proving, Bill told me, it is only necessary to avoid unsupervised repetition of a dose of any remedy with a potency higher than 12C. That's why most beginner home remedy kits include nothing stronger. The simple rule of thumb: take only one dose and see what happens. If it helps but the affliction remains or returns, you can cautiously take a second dose. If the first dose either cures or has no effect, take no more.

I soon had occasion to test that rule. When I returned to the mainland my left shoulder was no better, so I called Bill. He took my case over the phone and gave me Calcerea sulphuricum. It didn't help, so when I went to see Roger Morrison with Deanne, I asked for his help. He briefly took my case and gave me Sulphur. And he suggested I visit Jonathan Mayhew, DC, a chiropractor/homeopath who was a member of the first graduating class of Hahnemann Medical School.

By now we lived in the forest on the west side of the Sierra. Jon practiced in nearby Placerville and Sacramento. A Tuberculinum like myself, tall lanky Jon prescribed three months of twice-weekly adjustments. His job, he said, would be to loosen the frozen shoulder. Mine was to vigorously stretch it against the limits every day.

There was only a month before our annual move to Echo for the summer, and I didn't relish leaving its tranquility twice a week to drive down to Placerville for treatment. So I vigorously stretched and strengthened my arm by working in the garden with a pick and shovel, skiing, splitting wood, swimming and paddling a raft. To Jon's amazement I regained full mobility in my shoulder in just a month and a half—half the time he'd predicted, demonstrating the efficacy of Roger's prescription: a combination of medicine and physical therapy. The remedy had apparently cut the healing time in half.

In June I was invited to captain a raft 225 miles through the Grand Canyon. With a hundred river miles still to go, a violent rapid folded the heavily-laden boat in two and an ice chest smashed down on my right foot. The sharp pain made me fear that a bone had been broken. First Mate Deanne, always ready with her kit, had a dose of Arnica 200 in my mouth within seconds. Then I was ordered to hang my foot over the side in the 45 degree water while she packed ice in a plastic bag to make a cold compress.

That night in camp on a riverbank sandbar, she washed the wounds with Hypericum and switched from oral Arnica to Bryonia, coating the unbroken skin on my foot with the Arnica gel that pharmacist Michael Quinn had give us to test. The next day I could hobble around without sharp pain as we packed the boats for another day of rapids. But three days later, still on the river, the foot was no better and Deanne gave me daily doses of Symphytum in case a bone was broken. But this time Knit Bone didn't help.

A week later, back in Jon's office for a final shoulder adjustment, I had him examine my foot. He found a dislocation, which he corrected. For awhile the foot was better, then I apparently hiked too far in the wilderness behind our cabin, and it resumed hurting. I tried to fix the dislocation the way Jon had showed me, but the pain refused to go away. I was beginning to worry about the foot's failure to heal because we had a series of juicy wilderness walks scheduled for the following week.

When I went back to Jon, he was pessimistic about my hiking plans. "Your foot is probably going to dislocate again if you keep hiking in rough country. To heal, I'm afraid, it needs a long rest—unless you give it some homeopathic help. Is it better with motion, after you're warmed up?"

"You're thinking Rhus tox, eh? Yes, it's better once it's loose, but after that proving last winter in Hawaii I'm scared of taking Rhus tox again. Maybe I'm hypersensitive? I don't want to go through all THAT again!"

"Don't worry. You won't have to. Just take one dose of 30C and see what happens. If it helps, don't take another until it wears off. Just pay attention to your body and take it one dose at a time."

I didn't have much choice. We were about to trade mountain cabins for a week and I was looking forward to hiking new trails. So I put Bill's rule to the test. That night Deanne gave me Rhus tox 30C as we packed for the move. The next day at Wrights Lake my foot was much worse. I walked with a painful limp, even on level pavement! I just hoped I was experiencing a healing crisis.

Apparently I was. The following day my foot was better than it had been since the accident. After one day of rest, we set off on a long hike. The foot held up. Despite continued abuse on rough trails and cross country scrambling, it continued to heal. Within a week all pain was gone. I never had to take a second dose of Rhus tox, and I was able to enjoy all the hiking we had planned.

Before the summer was over, Deanne's hiking plans were also threatened by injury. Two days before a long awaited walk in Yosemite, she awoke with a painfully twisted right knee. It hurt with every step. A quick dose of Arnica 200 stopped the pain. Then she switched to Bryonia for two days while locally applying Arnica gel ... the same prescription that had first helped my foot. By the morning of our long walk, her knee was fully recovered.

I'm not the only family member to suffer from shoulder trouble. We were visiting my 85-year old father, Richard, and noticed him massaging his shoulder as we talked. He told us he had an injured rotator cup. Dr. Deanne immediately took his case and gave him Arnica 200 for the pain ... and my old friend Rhus tox to take later. She left him enough medicine to last several days, with instructions to call Michael Quinn at the Pharmacy for more if it worked. Dad reported an immediate fifty percent improvement, allowing him to give up the dozen aspirins he'd been taking for pain every day. Michael now keeps him supplied with remedies by mail.

Speaking of Michael, his Pharmacy has moved downstairs into the Clinic's Greek Temple to make more room for physicians upstairs.

To further her homeopathic education, Deanne journeyed to Boston in the summer of 1990 to take the NCH's most advanced course for lay practitioners. She plans to offer her own introductory courses on homeopathic self home care, and she hopes to open a modest practice for treatment of acute conditions.

That same summer Bill Gray and Vicky Menear moved their practice to the sleepy bedroom community of nearby Concord (see Homeopathic Sources) to reduce their work load. Bill sees the move as "an expansion, a branching out of Bay Area homeopathy" that will make room for new homeopaths at the Clinic while allowing him more time for writing and teaching. He'll continue to devote himself to the College he helped found in Hahnemann Clinic.

Bill promises to practice at least three days a week in Concord, continuing to accept new chronic cases. As part of peristroika, he's the first American homeopath to be invited to teach in Russia, where he hopes to launch a classical movement. And he plans to be part of the International School being organized in Europe by his old friend and teacher, George Vithoulkas. And he'll continue to lecture worldwide.

In the meantime, business at the Clinic has been steadily increasing as word rapidly spreads of the wonders that homeopathy can confer. As Bill put it, "Homeopathy holds the answer for the vast majority of chronic disease sufferers." And it's just as good at curing the common ailments we encounter every day.

So, why not consider it for yourself and your family? There's nothing to lose except your pain and discomfort. And there's everything to gain ... even happiness! The section on Homeopathic Sources that follows will get you pointed toward dependable help.

Homeopathic Sources

The following brief listings are recommended sources for physicians, organizations, remedies, books, tapes, general information, professional training, remedy kits ... anything and everything homeopathic.

Hahnemann Medical Clinic, 1918 Bonita Ave., Berkeley CA 94704, (415) 849–1925. At publication time, rates were as follows: initial constitutional visits: $300 for Bill Gray and Roger Morrison, $200 for the other 6 homeopaths; initial visit for a child: $115/hour; 45 minute visits are $84; half-hour acute visits or constitutional follow-ups are $60.

The Clinic provides ongoing courses in homeopathy, ranging from public introductory lectures for patients and prospective patients (at which questions may be asked), to the curriculum of Hahnemann College of Homeopathic Medicine for medical professionals.

Hahnemann Pharmacy, 1918 Bonita Ave., Berkeley, CA 94704, (415) 548–5015. Proprietor Michael Quinn supplies potent but safe remedies to fill the Clinic's prescriptions, as well as OTC remedies, kits, tapes and books.

Homeopathic Educational Services, 2124 Kittredge St., Berkeley, CA. 94704. (415) 653–9270. Proprietor-author Dana Ullman sells remedies, kits, tapes, books and a wide range of homeopathic information. Send a self-addressed stamped envelope to request an introductory or comprehensive catalog.

Organizations

National Center for Homeopathy, 1500 Massachusetts Ave., NW, Suite #42, Washington, D.C. 20005. (202) 223–6182. Dues of $35 yearly include the monthly newsletter, *Homeopathy Today.* The NCH sponsors conferences, provides public information and training for health professionals. Call or write for the names of classical homeopaths in your area.

International Foundation for Homeopathy, 2366 Eastlake Ave. E., #301, Seattle, WA 98102. (206) 324–8230. Dues of $25 yearly include the bi-monthly newsletter *Resonance.* The IFH also sponsors conferences and trains health professionals. Call or write for the names of classical homeopaths in your area.

Homeopathic Academy of Naturopathic Physicians, 11231 SE Market St., Portland, OR 97216. (503) 829–7326. Subscription to the HANP quarterly newsletter, *Simillimum* is $15.

American Institute of Homeopathy (same address and phone as the National Center) An organization composed exclusively of homeopathic MD's and dentists, it publishes the *Journal of the American Institute of Homeopathy*.

Homeopathic Books

The following are books that Dr. Deanne and I personally recommend from our limited reading. I'm sure there are many more fine ones that we have yet to discover. Listings are alphabetical, by author.

Boericke's—*Pocket Manual of Materia Medica with Repertory.* A compact, inexpensive, easy-to-use Materia Medica. Ideal for the serious home prescriber.

Coulter, Catherine R.—*Portraits of Homoeopathic Medicines.* Two separate volumes of psychophysical analyses of selected constitutional types. Delightful reading.

Coulter, Harris L.—*Homeopathic Medicine.* The "orange book" of chapter one provides an erudite, concise medical historian's view of the divine science.

Cummings, Stephen & Ullman, Dana—*Everybody's Guide to Homeopathic Medicine.* Ideal for the budding home prescriber with kit—along with Dr. Panos's book.

Garrett, Ray & Stone, Teresa—*Catching Good Health With Home-*

opathic Medicine. Featuring 75 pages of briefly told cured cases (often Bill Gray's) in the patient's own moving words.

Hubbard-Wright, Elizabeth—*A Brief Study Course in Homeopathy.* Remedy relationships and other tips not found elsewhere. For the home prescriber.

Kent, James Tyler—*Lectures on Homeopathic Philosophy.* Brilliant, insightful writing by the American master.

Panos, Maesimund & Heimlich, Jane—*Homeopathic Medicine at Home.* Ideal for the budding home prescriber with kit, along with the Cummings-Ullman book.

Pitcairn, Richard H. & Susan Pitcairn—*Natural Health for Dogs and Cats.* Taking care of your pet non-toxically. Includes birds, hamsters, rabbits, etc.

Shadman, Alonzo—*Who Is Your Doctor and* Why? Delightful, free-swinging critical comparison of homeopathy and allopathy by a homeopath-surgeon-hospital owner from Boston with 50 years healing experience.

Sheppard, Dorothy—*Homeopathy for the First-Aider.* An anecdote-filled how-to by a World War II lady British Medical officer ... with data not found elsewhere.

Ullman, Dana—*Homeopathy: Medicine for the 21st Century.* A comprehensive, up-to-date homeopathic text.

Vithoulkas, George—*Homeopathy: Medicine of the New Man.* The "blue book" from chapter one, a clear, fast-moving survey of the subject by the Greek Master. Ideal introduction to homeopathy.

Vithoulkas, George—*The Science of Homeopathy.* THE textbook and inspiration to outsiders ... especially discontent MD's who genuinely want to heal. The book's first section is condensed to form chapter 13.

Weiner, Michael & Goss, Kathleen—*The Complete Book of Homeopathy.* A clear, concise introduction.

Homeopaths Prominently Mentioned

Peggy Chipkin, F.N.P., Nancy Herrick, P.A., Roger Morrison, M.D. Jonathan Shore, M.D. and Matt Vuksinich, M.D., are all practitioners at Hahnemann Medical Clinic, 1918 Bonita Ave., Berkeley, CA 94704.

Bill Gray, M.D. & Vicky Menear, M.D.
2108 Grant St.
Concord, CA 94520

Linda Johnston, M.D.
14624 Sherman Way #404
Van Nuys, CA 91405

Jonathan Mayhew, D.C. (our doc in Placerville. See Epilogue)
681 Main St. #212, Placerville, CA 95667 and
4096 Bridge St. (A), Fair Oaks, CA 95628

Richard Moskowitz, M.D. (Vaccination, Chapter 16)
Turning Point Family Wellness Center
173 Mt. Auburn St.
Watertown, Mass. 02172

Richard H. Pitcairn, D.V.M. (Kids and Dogs, Chapter 14)
1283 Lincoln Ave.
Eugene, Oregon 97401

Mark Rosen, D.O.
655 Homer Ave.
Palo Alto, CA 95301

Michael Traub, N.D. (Kids and Dogs ... our Doc in Hawaii)
75–5759 Kuakini Highway #202
Kailua-Kona, HI 96740

About the Author

Growing up in Berkeley, Robert S. Wood obtained a B.S. from U.C. in 1952 before taking an editorial job in a San Francisco publishing house. He has since served as staff Correspondent for *Time*, *Life*, *Sports Illustrated* and *Wilderness Camping* and contributed to *Outside*, *Sierra*, *The New York Times* and other magazines.

After fortunate investments permitted early retirement from journalism, he devoted his time to wilderness and foreign travel, river rafting, hiking and personal growth—and writing books about his adventures. Sales of his first six books approach 200,000 copies.

He now divides his year—with wife Deanne and daughter Angela (Gellie)—between homes in the Sierra foothills and Hawaii, and a mountain cabin on the edge of Desolation Wilderness. With Deanne he continues to indulge his Tuberculinum yen for travel. At present he's completing a book on dayhiking before beginning another on homeopathy.

Between trips, Deanne teaches elementary school and introductory courses in homeopathy, while continuing to treat her friends and family homeopathically.